The Christian Men's Midlife Fitness Primer

By Dave Yarnell

http://Christianiron.com

The Christian Men's Midlife Fitness Primer

Written by Dave Yarnell, Christianiron.com

Forward

Is it sinful to be fabulously fit, super strong, or possess a great physique as a middle-aged Christian man? Seems like a silly question, doesn't it?

Well, if it's not a sin, why do so few Christian men (or women) fall into any of these above categories? Perhaps there is no single answer to this question, but there are several possibilities.

For one, **we Christians do like to eat when we have social gatherings**. Potluck suppers, pre and post service buffets, snacks at bible studies, etc. To make matters worse, I have not seen too many healthy foods at these gatherings. It's usually "comfort foods". Also, while most Christians adhere to the part of the Bible that tells us to refrain from drinking too much strong drink (many abstain altogether), **somehow we overlook the passages about gluttony being a sin as well.**

"For bodily exercise profits a little, but godliness is profitable for all things, having promise of the life that now is and of that which is to come". 1Tim 4:8

Paul talked about **physical exercise being of a little value, while spiritual exercise is of a great value**. Note that he did not say physical exercise was worthless! I would concur that the soul is of far more value than the body, but that is no justification for completely neglecting the body, as many of our ilk are guilty.

After all, the body is the temple of the Holy Spirit, so we need to take care of it as such, right?

"Do you not know that your body is the temple of the Holy Spirit [who is] in you, whom you have from God, and you are not your own?" 1Cor 6:19

"For you were bought at a price; therefore glorify God in your body and in your spirit, which are God's." 1Cor 6:20

To be sure, we must keep things in balance. **Working out for countless hours, 6 or 7 days a week is likely to take away time from more important things like spending time with family, in church, our jobs, etc.** Unfortunately though, some use this as an excuse not to workout at all.

I propose that any exercise is way better than none. I think if we are all honest with ourselves, we can find some time to workout. How much time is spent watching TV?

How much time pursuing sedentary hobbies? Maybe we are workaholics. The list goes on. **The point is this; stop making excuses and start moving!**

The disciples and great men of the Bible did not go to World Gym or Bally's, or any gym, you might say. True enough, but they also didn't sit in front of a computer all day, and then get in their car and drive home so they could sit in front of the TV while other devices did the wash, dishes, etc, either.

In biblical times, people walked everywhere, rowed boats when they went fishing, had to manually carry buckets of water from the well to wherever, and did wash by hand. There was little need for barbells or treadmills as there is today.

We also need to address the way society views the Christian man of today. **We are often viewed as wimps, geeks, not masculine, and soft.**

John Eldridge speaks of Christians being compared to Mr. Rogers

Don't get me wrong, he's a great guy, but may not be the epitome of the Christian warrior

Was Samson a pencil neck? How about young David when he slew Goliath, Was he a nerd? Was Jesus acting wimpy when he overturned the tables of the money changers and drove them out of the temple? Were James and John not called the sons of thunder? I could go on, but I think you get the point.

Maybe if more of us could bench press 300 pounds, or compete in a triathlon, or looked like we were chiseled out of stone, we'd get a little more respect! (Not that the respect of the world is our primary concern). But maybe you have no aspiration to be superman. Perhaps you just need to lose a little weight or gain some muscle tone, or be able to run around the block without keeling over.

Whichever category you find yourself in, I 'm sure I can offer some ideas here that will help you reach your goal, and maybe even set some tougher goals for yourself in the future.

The LORD will give strength to His people; The LORD will bless His people with peace.Ps29:11

Chapter 1

Where Do I Start?

Blessed [is] the man whose strength [is] in You, Whose heart [is] set on pilgrimage. Ps 84:5

As in any other endeavor in life, **in order to reach a goal, we must first clearly define that goal; otherwise, we'll just be wandering in the wilderness" for years,** and will likely never see the Promised Land. I won't tell you what your goals should be, that is up to you. **I will suggest that you don't set them too high or too low.**

While you should have a long term goal in mind, you also need to **set some realistic short term goals that will stack victory on top of victory until the ultimate goal is reached**. This is not to imply that you won't ever fail. You will! Greatness has seldom, if ever, been achieved by anyone without overcoming failures.

When a baby is learning to walk, does he just get up and start walking right away? No, he falls down over and over, but **he keeps getting back up and trying, and guess what?**

Eventually he's walking like a champ, even running, skipping, jumping. Be persistent! I assure you, it will pay off down the road

You must reasonably evaluate how much time you are willing to spend in pursuit of your goal (s), as part of setting that goal. For example, to say "I want to be Mr. Olympia in 2 years, and I will devote 15 minutes a day, 3 days a week, to that end" is simply ridiculous.

If you said "I'd like to lose maybe 10 pounds of fat, and gain 5 pounds of muscle in the next year", then that 15 minutes 3 times a week might just be reasonable. You would really have to bust your butt for those 15 minutes, and that would not include some warm-up time, but it's feasible.

Even a lofty goal, such as becoming a competitive power lifter, does not require the amount of time that you might imagine. Sure, you could do 3 hour workouts 6 days a week in pursuit of that goal, but in doing so, you'd most likely do more harm than good.

There are guys that some call "**gym rats**", who spend long hours in the gym and make minimal progress. They socialize, discuss the virtues of the latest article in a men's fitness magazine, what the hot supplements are.

They dress the part, and seek the advice of the personal trainer that looks like he never did a hard day's work in his life, in or out of the gym.

You could pick up a copy of one of the popular body-building magazines and try to emulate the workout of one of the stars therein, but if you don't use steroids and/or growth hormone and/or every nutritional supplement that comes down the pike, you might kill yourself, or at least burnout in short order and quit.

I'll be honest with you here. Yes, I have used steroids in my life, and yes, they work. I can also honestly tell you that almost 20 years after I took my last pill or injection of "the juice", I have matched my best ever bench press done on the juice, and come very near my best ever deadlift on the stuff, and all this as a much older and busier man.

I am not out to blow my own horn here. I am far from being God's gift to the fitness world. I am not particularly genetically gifted; I am just trying to tell you that if I can do it, anyone who sets their mind to it can also do it. **Learn from your mistakes; don't be discouraged if you miss a weight, a rep, a lap or a workout. Keep a positive attitude, be persistent, never give up, and YOU WILL BE REWARDED!!!!!**

Chapter 2

Keeping a Training log or Journal

A wise man [is] strong, Yes, a man of knowledge increases strength*; Prov24:5*

I can not over emphasize this point. You MUST keep track of your training in order to know if you are progressing according to plan.

The **more details you retain, the better.** I simply have an excel spreadsheet on which I put workout day/date across the top, filling in sets, reps, weights, even comments about how I was feeling on a given day, what vitamins I took, etc.

You can refer back to this log and see clearly when and where you have progressed well, or progress has stopped, or you have gone backwards (eeek!)

If you are trying to gain or lose weight, it would be a **good idea to keep a diet journal, as well.** You don't have to count every calorie you consume, but a general idea of what you ate, how much, how it affected your day or your workout, and a daily or at least 2 or 3 times a week scale reading would be helpful.

Keep in mind, though, that **the scale reading is not the be-all, end-all.** You could be losing fat and gaining muscle at the same time (isn't that special!!) This would mean you're shaping up very well, yet the scale would not show it too much.

Body mass index is a heavily used indicator, but a tape measure, scale, mirror and seeing your strength increases in your journal are all good also.

Use a composition book, a computer, a notebook, whatever you like, but do it!

Chapter 3

Should I join a gym?

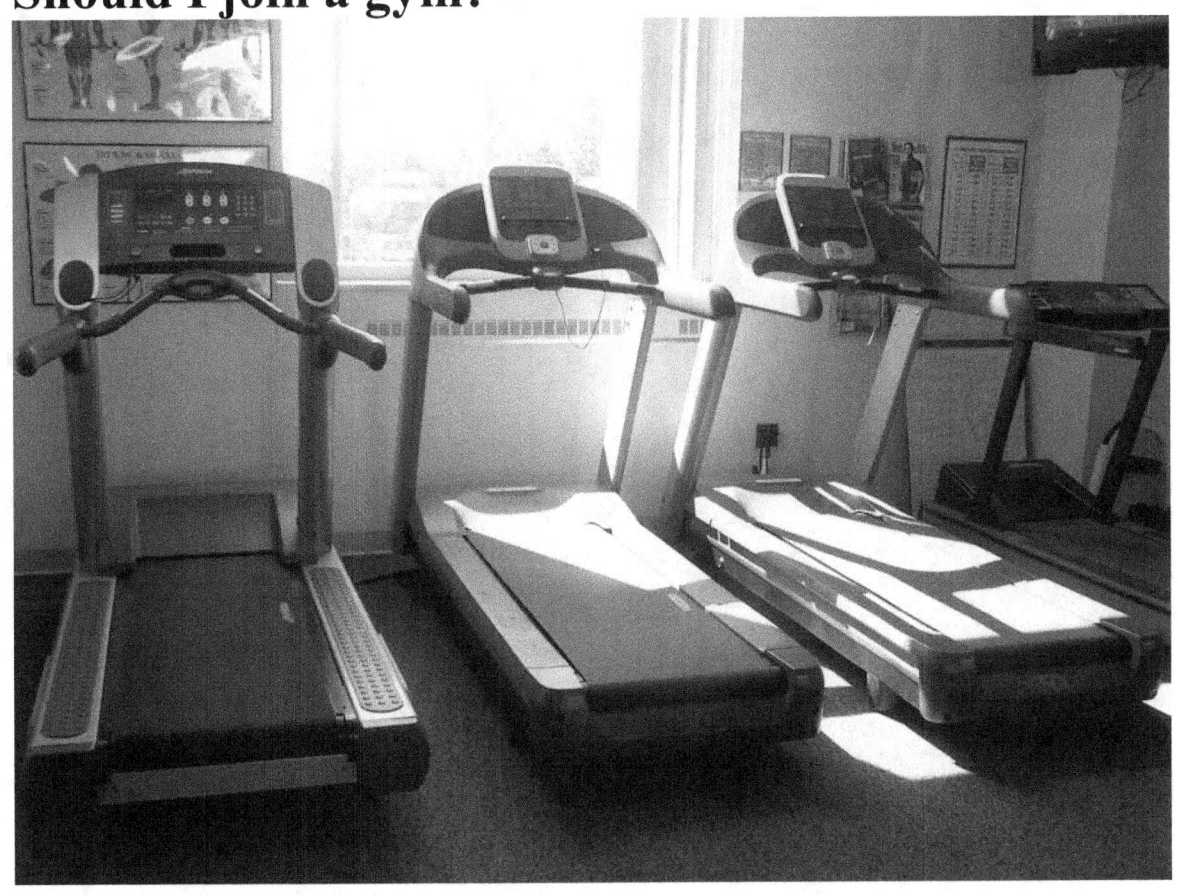

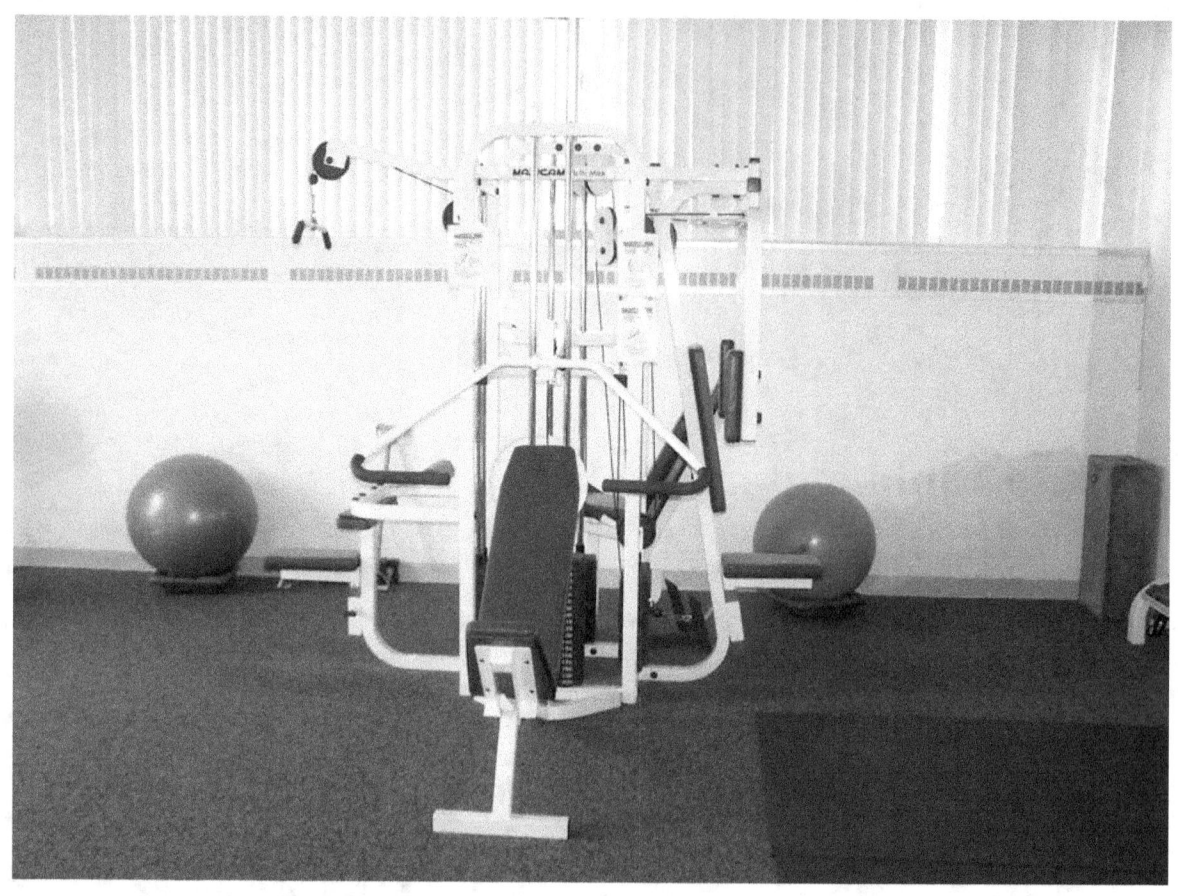

Many a commercial gym operation has gotten rich off the backs of out of shape folks who **get bullied into long term contracts because they feel the need to make a commitment**. You will have made a financial commitment, to be sure, but that may not be enough to keep you going to the gym for the duration of your time commitment. **People who sign up for a multiyear contract and then quit after a few weeks or months are a commercial gym's best friends.**

With that being said, many gyms have a good variety of good equipment that runs the gamut from cardio to free weights, and various isolation type machines. They may also have steam, sauna, swimming pools and other nice amenities.

A word about steam & saunas

These are one of the very beneficial amenities available at many gyms and fitness centers.

Just sitting in one of these accelerates your heart rate thereby increasing metabolic rate and burning more calories. Sweating profusely is also a great way to rid the body of toxins that might not be removed from other bodily functions as readily.

There are some "detox" programs which call for spending hours each day in saunas, along with diets that are "clean", meaning organic and hopefully free of toxins and chemicals.

Other such programs call for eliminating wastes in a more traditional fashion, but using "colonics" and/or avoiding solid foods and consuming lots of broths, soups and other liquids.

While this may seem uncomfortable or even gross to some, the benefits obtained may just be worth the effort and trouble.

Many of the "diet" books I have seen lately suggest using a dry sauna several times a week or more to enhance weight loss efforts.

Why sauna? Dry heat is preferable, many doctors say, as steam often contains chlorine from the water supply, which itself is considered toxic to the body, especially at higher levels. I have even read that taking hot showers for long periods can cause over-exposure to chlorine unless you have well water or proper filtration.

If you can afford the several hundred (and up) per year membership fees, don't mind working out where others can see and hear you, then by all means, join a gym.

If you do, though, **don't get caught up in the socialization game to the point where you are not concentrating on your workout.** Now don't get me wrong, you don't have to be an ignorant zombie, never interacting with others, etc. In fact, it's good to develop some relationships with other folks who have similar goals, and **one should always use a "spotter" when lifting heavy weights in certain free weight lifts.**

A little good spirited competition between you and a peer or 2 could be just what the doctor ordered to keep things fun in the gym and that is one of the keys to staying with it.

Also, beware gym owners and personal trainers who give you some arbitrary program that does not take your skills (or lack thereof), body type, or personal goals in mind when coming up with the workout scheme. Of course, if you don't know how to use a particular machine or a free weight exercise, get someone in the know to show you how.

Chapter 4

What are the alternatives?

There are **plenty of viable alternatives to joining a gym**, contrary to what that XYZ Fitness sales person will tell you. You could build your own home gym (this could get expensive). You could do pure bodyweight exercises that require no equipment. You could make your own equipment and use it at home or on your own property. **You could walk, jog, run, bicycle, and any number of other things that are essentially free and that you set your own schedule for.** You could buy the latest gadget or gizmo that you've seen on an infomercial touted by some "fitness guru" or the other. In the short term, you could sign up for some boot-camp that's designed to whip you into shape fast, but requires a serious time and/or financial commitment.

Confused enough yet? Sorry, that is not my intent. Let's face facts. I like pumping iron, so I workout with free weights for the most part, sometimes at home, sometimes in a gym. You might find that boring, or it might not suit your needs. I could tell you if you don't do what I do, you're wasting your time.

I've read many a "fitness expert" book or forum, etc. in which the writer touts his way as the only way, everyone else is wrong, any other program is useless, and so forth.

While you and I know there is only one true way to salvation, this is just not true with fitness!

If you are starting at ground zero, than just about any of the above methods or equipment will have some beneficial outcome. The real key is to find something you actually enjoy doing, and this may take some experimentation.

One caveat here; **if something sounds too good to be true, it probably is**. There is no magic bullet. There is no secret exercise or one device that you can do for 30 seconds a day and get real results.

There are many devices sold which make claims to be the last piece of exercise equipment you'll ever need. Not likely! I won't say all of these things are worthless.

Some actually work fairly well. You will probably need several of these devices to get even a decent overall workout, and if you get beyond the novice level of training, you will likely outgrow these quickly.

Again, if you want to go ahead and try one of these, go ahead. It won't hurt you (unless used incorrectly).

Most of these devices emulate an exercise you could do without the device. It may make it more comfortable to perform, but probably is not necessary.

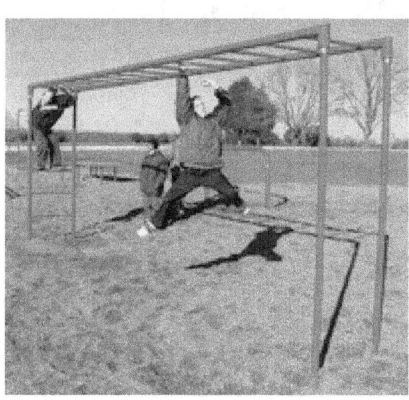

Above is shown an outdoor gym with monkey bars, etc. These are usually found in public parks and recreation centers, and are free to use by anyone. This type of equipment/workout is one of the alternatives to joining a gym.

☺

Below is shown one of the old school pieces of apparatus that can be used as an all-around fitness tool, is relatively cheap, and will yield some results for those who use diligently. This is yet another alternative to gym membership.

There are actually website forums dedicated to the use of these, and there are some newer models which provide considerably more challenging tension than its original version.

This is a nice piece of easy to use, portable equipment with which you can get a quick, decent workout anywhere, anytime.

Bullworker®

FULL RANGE

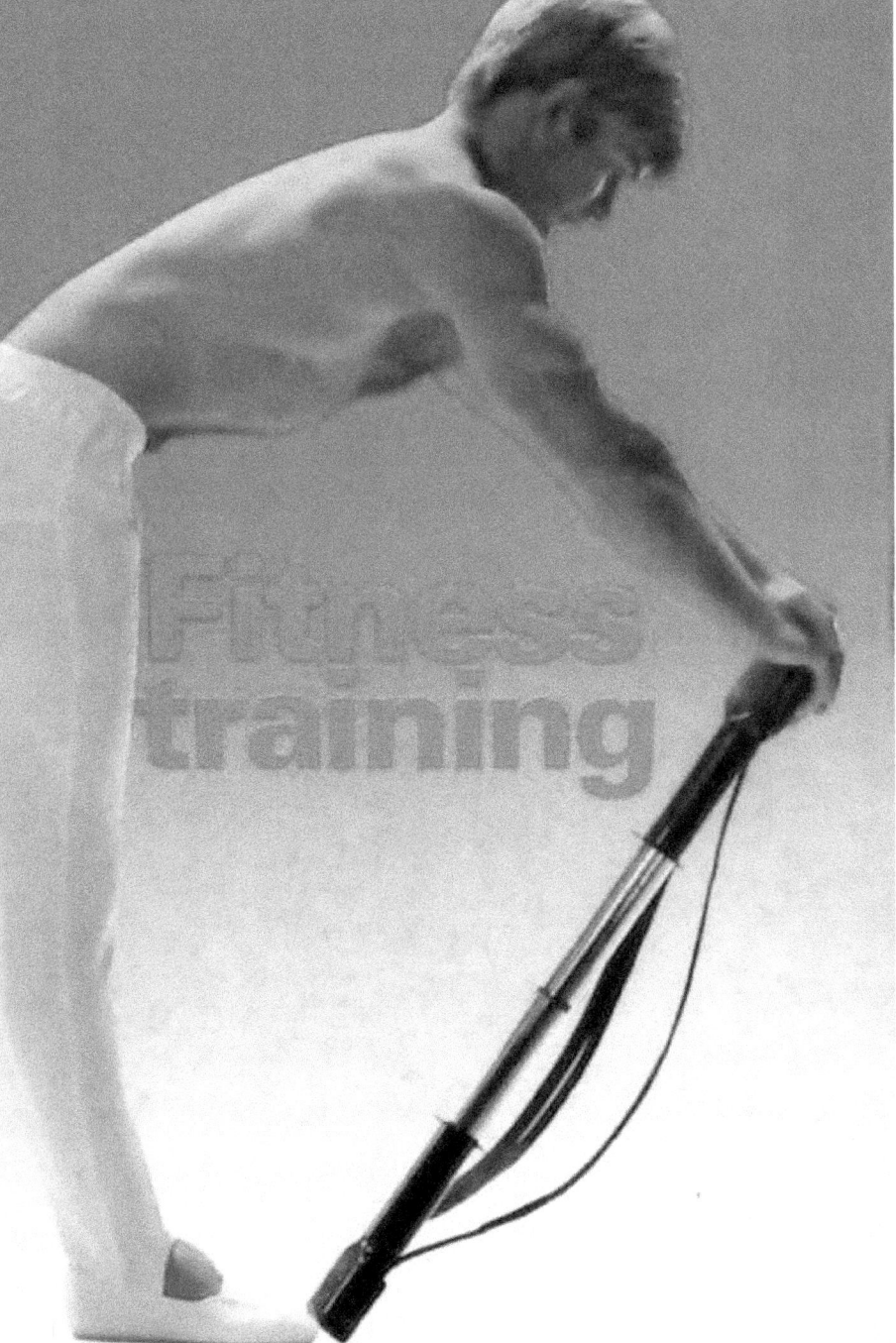

Fitness
training

I happen to have owned one of these before I started weight training, and still own one today.

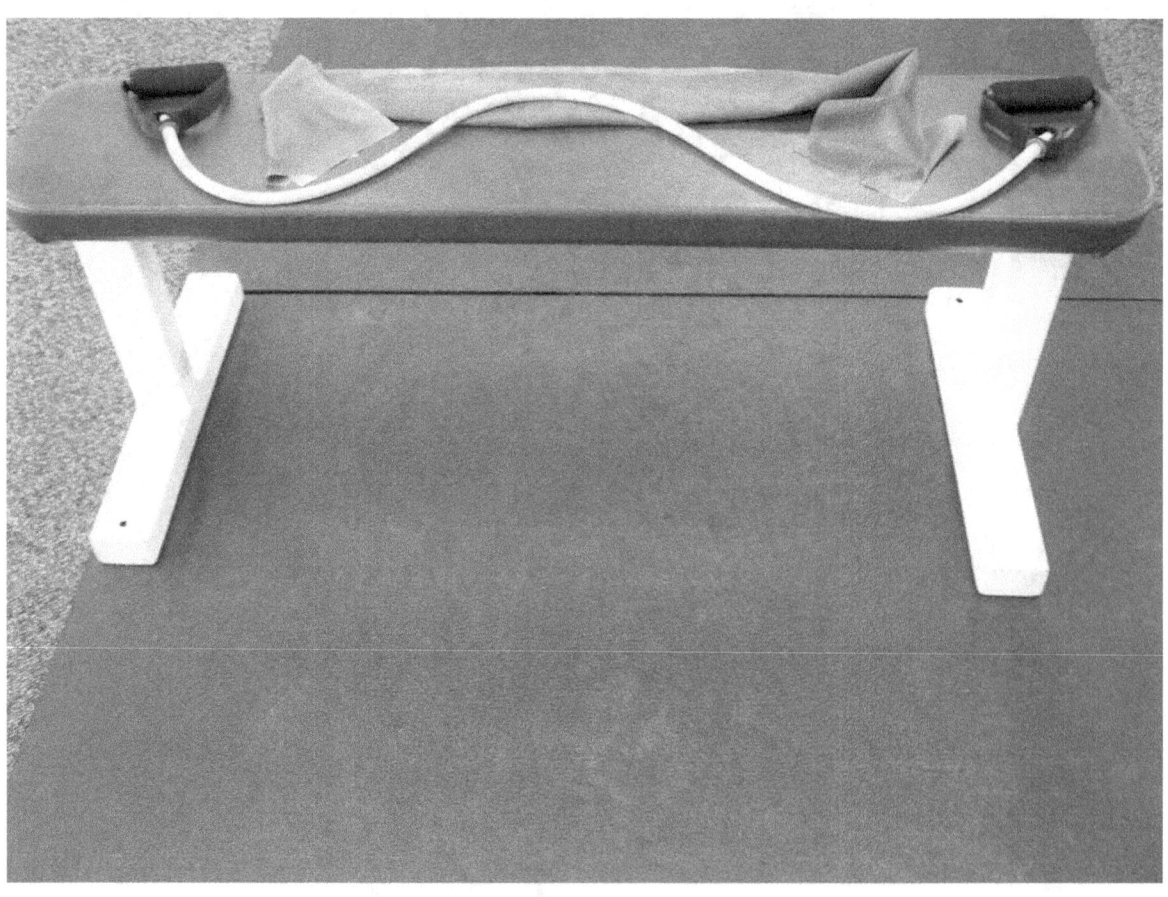

Pilate's style bands and Tubing above

These are inexpensive, very portable and can provide enough resistance to add some challenge to an otherwise boring free
Style workout (bodyweight only)

Δ

Below is shown a piece of equipment to assist with abdominal crunches

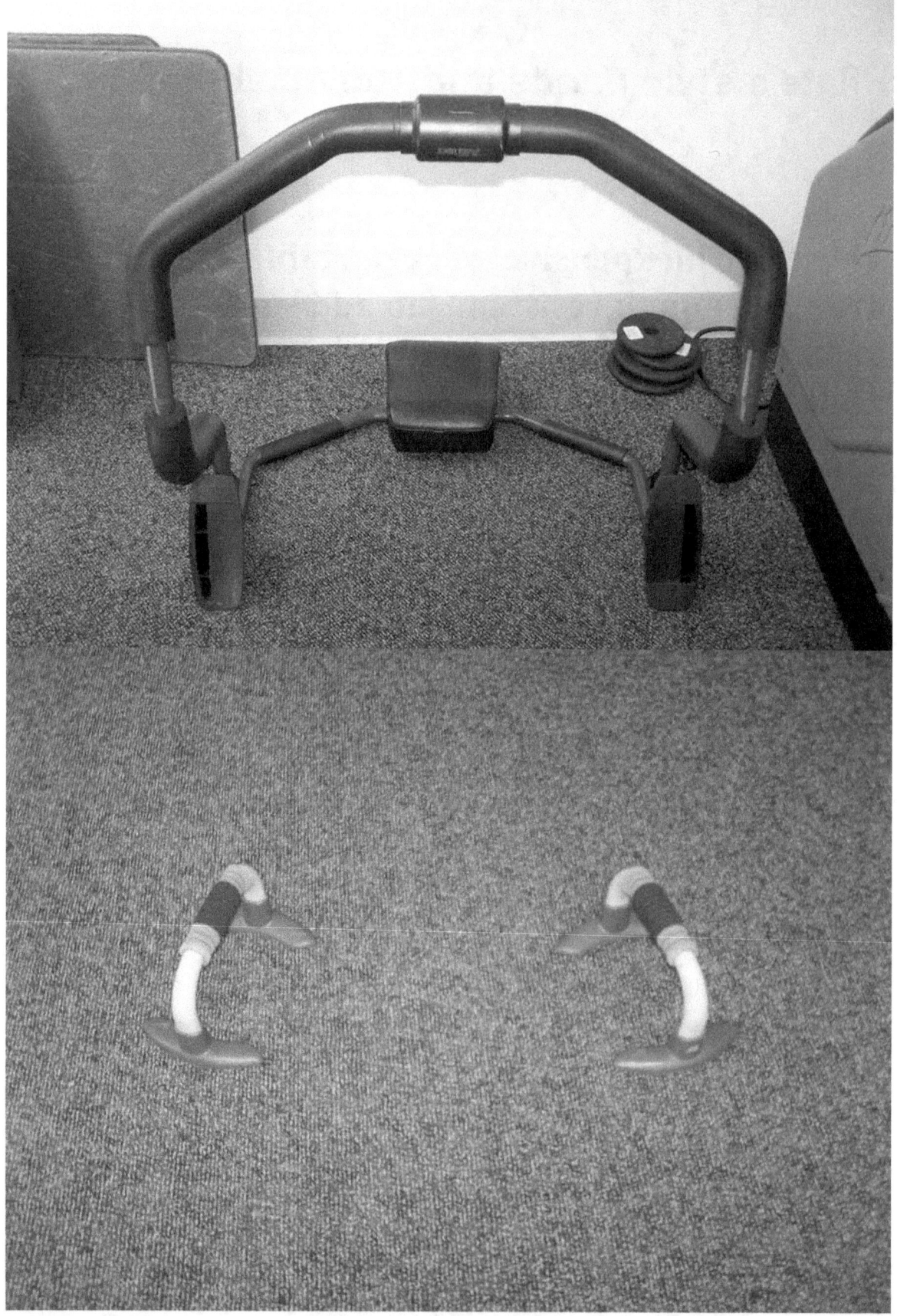

These items (above) are pushup handles.

These enable more range of motion and angle variations on the original equipment-free version of the pushup.
These have been touted as able to facilitate the best upper body workouts possible.
While pushups have always been and continue to be one of the best non-weight lifting upper body movements you could do, and these might even make them a little better, the purveyors of these devices may just be pushing it a wee bit.

♥

Below you see a flying saucer looking device known to fitness buffs as a Bosu ball.

It is really more like half a ball, as you can see. This is a variation of the stability ball which has become all the rage on the fitness circuit lately. Doing pushups on the Bosu ball, standing on the ball while performing other exercises, add an extra degree of difficulty to a movement.

This calls into play more core strength and balancing ability. It improves agility as well.

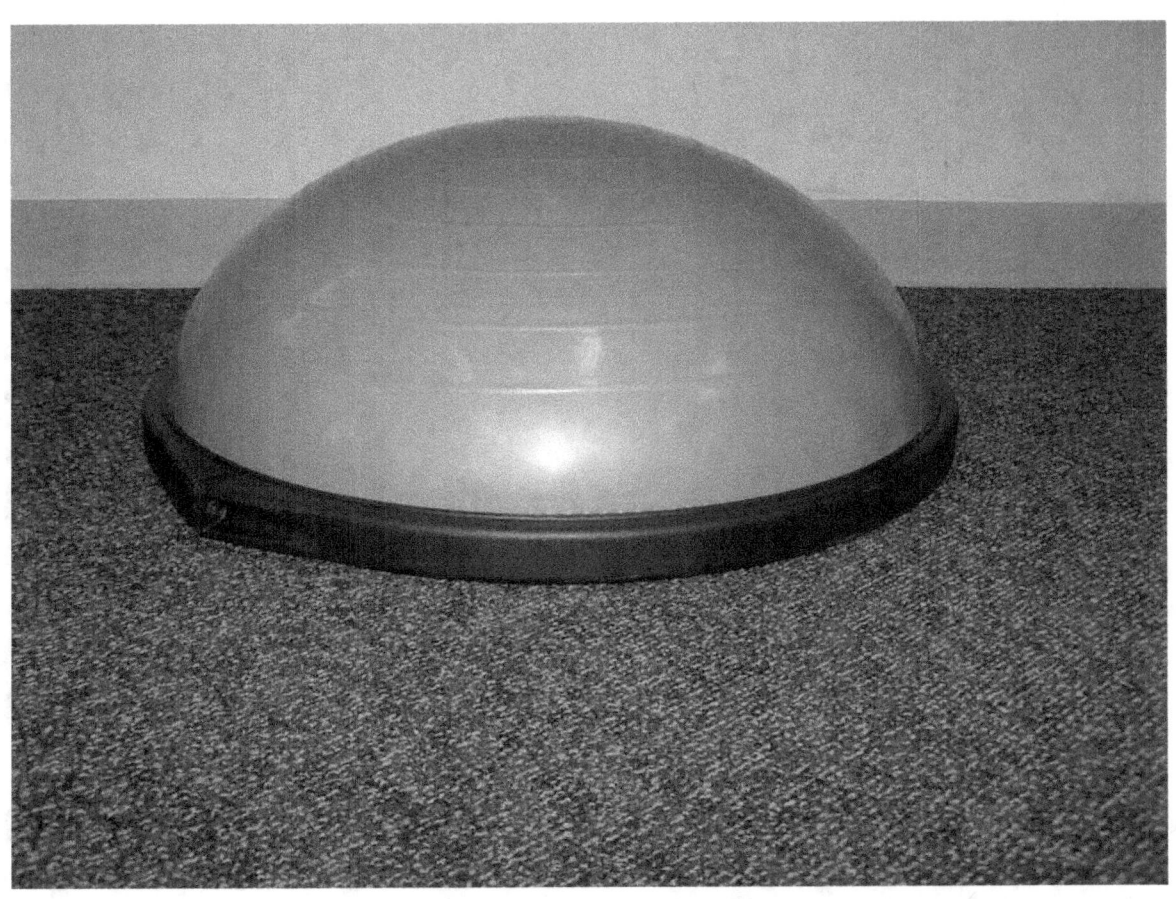

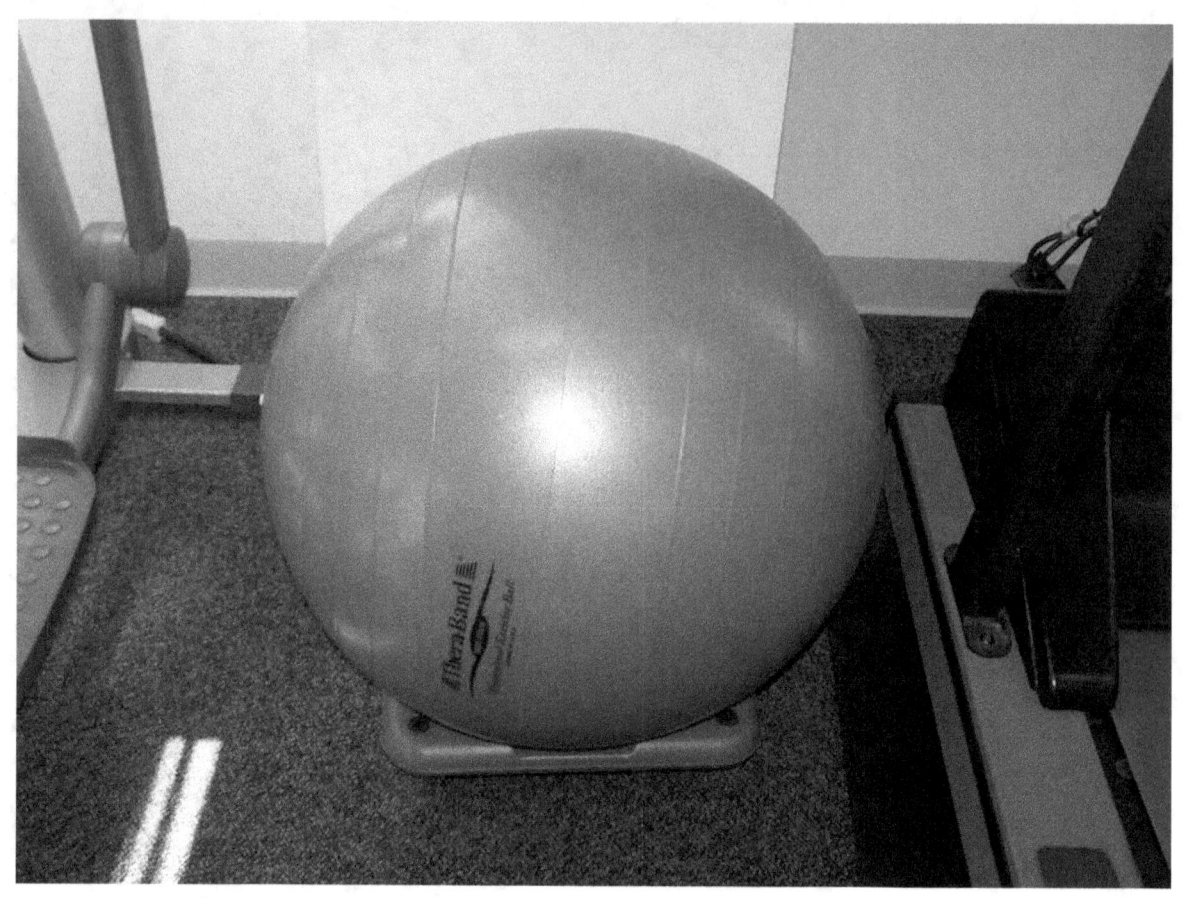

Above is shown the stability ball

These balls are used for many core and abdominal exercises, but can be used as part of any routine for any body part.

Again, they add difficulty in requiring balance, agility and core strength. Trying to maintain one's stability on the ball while performing a movement adds the extra impact.

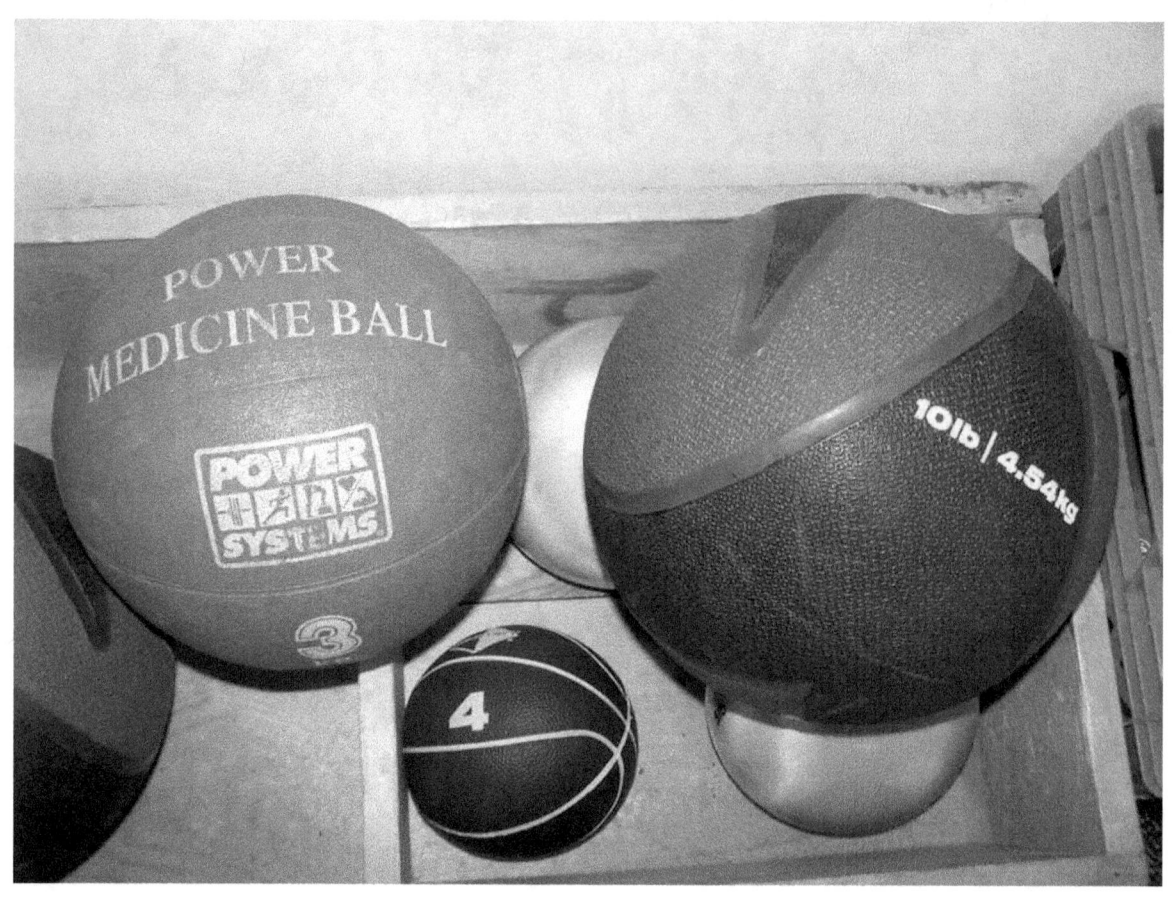

Above we see a few "Medicine Balls"

These are weighted balls used to create a workout from a simple game of catch, or train your abs by sitting back to back with a partner and passing the ball back and forth in a circular fashion.

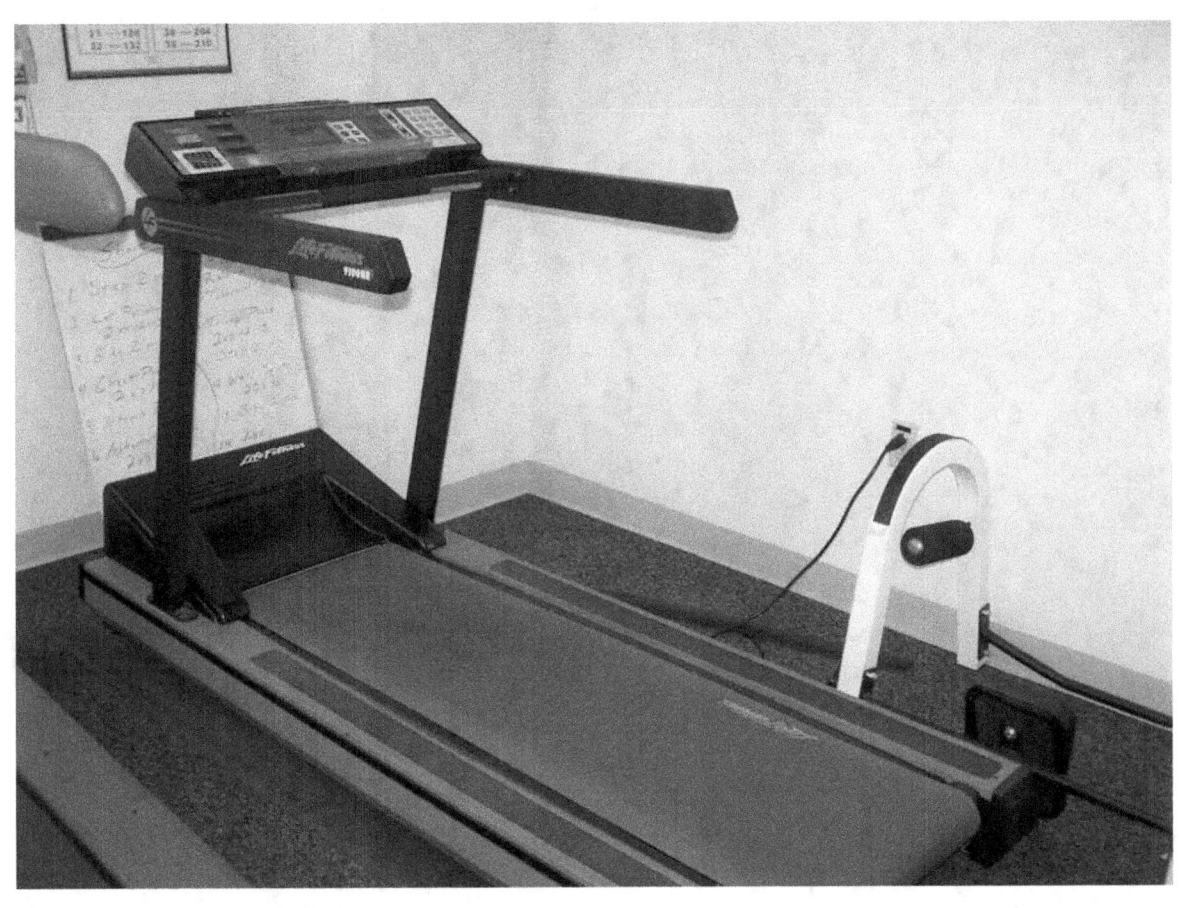

Of course, many folks choose to buy a treadmill as the primary or only piece of home gym equipment

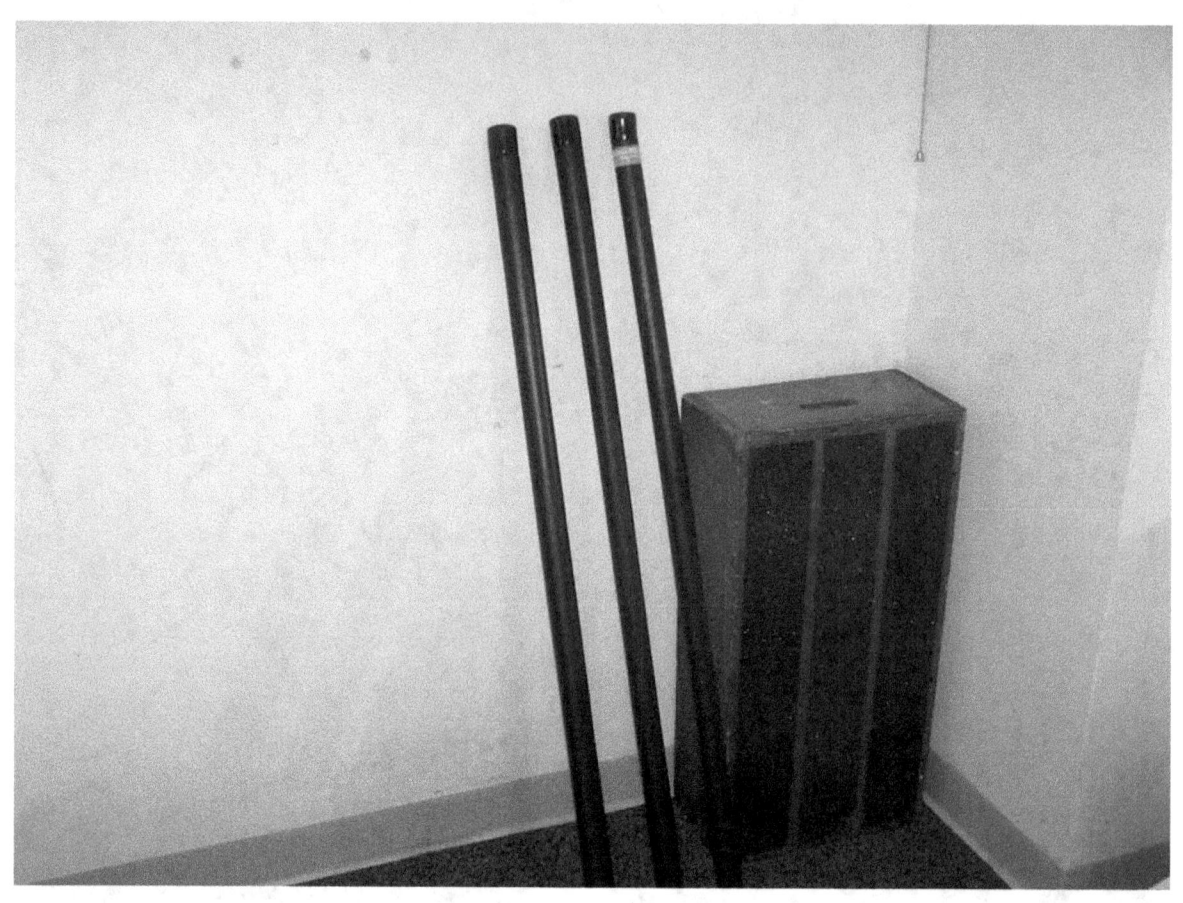

Here you see weighted "Body bars" and a small "Plyo-box"

Body bars are soft and can be used to do any traditional weight-lifting style movement with a little more comfort. They can also be used for abdominal twists and the like to add difficulty over doing free style or with a broom handle.

The Plyo-box is used for stepping up onto or down from when doing aerobic style workouts, or one could just jump on and off with force. The one shown is short. Serious Plyometrics work requires taller boxes, generally.

Chapter 5

How do I choose?

I can really only give some guidelines on this. **If you to want gain muscle size and/or strength, then riding a bike or jogging is not going to cut the mustard.**

If you need to lose a lot of fat, doing a heavy free weight program is not going to quite fit the bill, at least not by itself. **You need to tailor the workout to your needs and goals.**

I'll give you some examples of what types of exercise may meet what type of goal:

Losing weight

Walking

Jogging

Running

Bike riding

Circuit weight training

Jumping rope

Using a hula hoop

Personal sized trampoline

Swimming laps

Walking in a pool

Using elliptical machine

Using stair stepper machine

Actually walking or running up and down stairs

Calisthenics

Interval training

High intensity interval training

Any combination of the above

Be creative!

Toning up, gaining strength without gaining much weight

Bodyweight exercises, I.E;

Pushups

Pull-ups

Squats

Bodyweight plus a little extra exercise
(I will give more details further on)

Calisthenics
Using resistance bands

Gaining real muscle mass and increasing strength

Lifting weights, primarily free weights

Using Plyometrics techniques

Sprinting

Doing "strongman" style moves
(More on this later)

Using bodyweight moves with added weight and/or making more difficult variations

Notice that some things fall under more than one heading, i.e. calisthenics, which is useful for both fat-burning and light muscle building.

Chapter 6

Nutrition

Acts 14:17

Nevertheless He did not leave Himself without witness, in that He did good, gave us rain from heaven and fruitful seasons, filling our hearts with food and gladness."

The first point I would like to make here is this; **stay away from fad diets.** Zero fat, zero carbohydrate, juice diets, salad only diets, etc. While **restrictive diets can help one to lose weight in the short term, they are not sustainable, and the dieter is likely to eventually gain back all the weight that was lost, and then some.**

Make small, steady improvements in your eating habits over time, stick to the changes, and the weight will come off, perhaps slowly, but surely.

There needs to be a **proper ratio of protein, carbohydrate and fats for a healthy diet.** If you train with weights, you will need more protein than the average person of your size and weight. If you are a distance runner, you will need a little more protein and considerably more carbohydrate than a sedentary person.

Eliminating fat altogether is unwise and unhealthy, but cutting down on saturated fats is desirable. You want the **correct ratio of HDL to LDL in the blood.** HDL is high density lipoproteins, while LDL is low density lipoproteins. When you get a routine physical from your doctor, usually this will come up on your blood work report along with cholesterol levels, etc.

Generally speaking, HDL is good, LDL is bad. **Using extra virgin olive oil in your cooking is a good step in the right direction.**

Generally, protein should compose about 25-30% of total diet, carbohydrate about 50-60%, and fat 20-25%. Experts disagree slightly on exact ratios for different folks, but if you workout the number I'm using should at least be in the ballpark for you.

There have been some books and sources recently suggesting that the old government pyramid diagram is too heavy on complex carbohydrates and not heavy enough on protein. The diagram came about at least partially trying to sway people away from protein sources that are also high in fat (whole milk products, red meat)

The sources mentioned seem to feel that protein is maligned by this concept only because of its being associated with these heart-unfriendly saturated fats. If you can stick to better protein sources, such as those found in packaged supplements or tuna, low fat cottage cheese, etc, and then upping the ratio of protein may not be a bad idea. Protein helps insulin regulation, has a higher "**thermic effect**" and makes you feel "fuller" when eaten.

The **thermic effect** has to do with the amount of calories it takes to process and digest protein. It takes considerably more calories than it does to digest fat or carbohydrates, thus another good benefit!

Carbohydrates should consist of mostly complex sources rather than simple carbohydrates (sugars).Whole grain pasta, whole grain breads, dark rice, potatoes, vegetables would fall in this class.

One of the catch phrases that have been bounced around a lot recently is "**Glycemic Index**" of carbohydrate food sources.

This has to do with how much sugar is in the food and how much of an insulin reaction that food causes.

More recently, nutritionists have been using a more accurate measure of this, which is called "**Glycemic load**".

Glycemic load takes into account the fiber and protein found in the food, which makes its absorption rate and metabolism different.

To simplify the concept, the more fiber a carbohydrate food contains, the slower it is absorbed, the fuller it makes you feel and the less of an insulin spike it creates.

Obviously, these are desirable qualities to a dieter.

This is one reason fiber supplementing has become more popular these days.

Of course, fiber also helps to maintain regularity, which is also vital to keeping the metabolism running smoothly.

Irregularity can cause toxins to be held in the body longer, not being flushed out as they should. This in turn can cause internal inflammation and also lead to more infection and illness as well as a slowed metabolism.

Inflammation can cause the energy machines known as mitochondria to not function as well, which contributes to poor metabolism, low energy levels, and weight gain and/or difficulty in losing weight.

Protein

Good sources of protein are tuna (packed in water, not oil, if using canned variety), chicken, turkey, lean red meat, other white fleshed fish like Pollock, etc. Salmon is also both high in protein as well as omega 3 fatty acids, which both provide energy and help to adjust HDL/LDL levels.

One word of caution on protein; many bodybuilders and lifters over do it in this department. The typical bodybuilding magazine will have numerous ads for protein supplements, and may suggest taking lots of extra protein, especially their particular brand. While hard training lifters definitely need more protein, double or triple the normal needs is not a good idea. **This puts an unnecessary load on your kidneys and digestive system, and excesses will end up being stored as fat, just as any other excess calories.**

If you are trying to lose weight, reduce overall calories and or burn some off. If you want to gain some muscle, increase caloric intake slightly, with the emphasis on quality protein and complex carbohydrates. Obviously, you must put in some weight training and/or hi-intensity bodyweight work to build muscle also.

In order to help you in your eating plan (I don't like to use the term diet), I am adding a list here of good foods and bad foods.

GOOD FOODS	BAD FOODS
Tuna, packed in water if canned (Protein)	anything fried
Turkey (Protein)	Cake, donuts, candy
Low fat cottage cheese (protein)	regular mayo
Oat meal (Complex carbs, some protein)	Sugary cereals
Whole grain breads, pasta (Complex carbs)	white bread
Colorful veggies (simple-complex carbs, vitamins)	white sugar
Fruits (good form of simple carbs, vitamins) cream	whole sour
Low fat or non-fat yogurt (simple carbs, some protein, Beneficial microorganisms	Ice cream
Low fat milk (protein)	chips, cheese doodles
Legumes, unsalted nuts (read labels)	gravies, sauces
Lean red meat, venison, buffalo (protein)	soda, juice with sugar added

Salmon, sardines (protein, omega-3's) filets   boxed, breaded fish

America's 10 most unwanted
Wanted: dead and gone!

1. white sugar, white bread, white rice, "wheat" flour products (Not Whole wheat)

2. trans fats

3. "hydrogenated" anything

4. soda

5. High Fructose Corn Syrup

6. High Glycemic index, low nutrition value Carbohydrates

7. "Low Carb" diets

8. Excessive Alcohol consumption

9. Ingestion/absorption of toxins

10. Sedentary lifestyle

This list is not all inclusive of every potentially negative thing you could eat, just some of the very worst.

I can't really over emphasize learning to **read and understand labels.**
The food industry stays "hip" with the latest diet trends and crazes and tries to appeal to the public by packaging and advertising their goods accordingly.
So many foods will highlight the phrase "low fat" on the front of the box, and the item truly is lower in fat.
However, **they often replace fat with sugar**, which may cause more harm to some than the fat did, especially diabetic or pre-diabetic folks.
Beware "High fructose corn syrup" which is often found in things we think are good for us, like some protein bars, for instance.
Many artificial sweeteners have been reported by some researchers to cause metabolic problems for users, especially when consumed in high, regular doses.
Diet soda is one area in which we can get into trouble with this.
People tend to think because something is labeled "sugar free" or low calorie, it is therefore safe to consume in mass quantities.
There is no "free lunch" The body does not handle non-nutritive chemicals and additives like it does the God-given food that does not come in a shiny, attractive package.
"Diet" soda is one of the biggest contributors to poor health and weight maintenance problems in our modern era.
Hydrogenated fats are another ugly part of modern mass produced foods. These are not recognized by the body as nutrition, because it really isn't.
The body can only handle so much of these kinds of things before it starts to break down and our health and fitness suffers greatly for it.

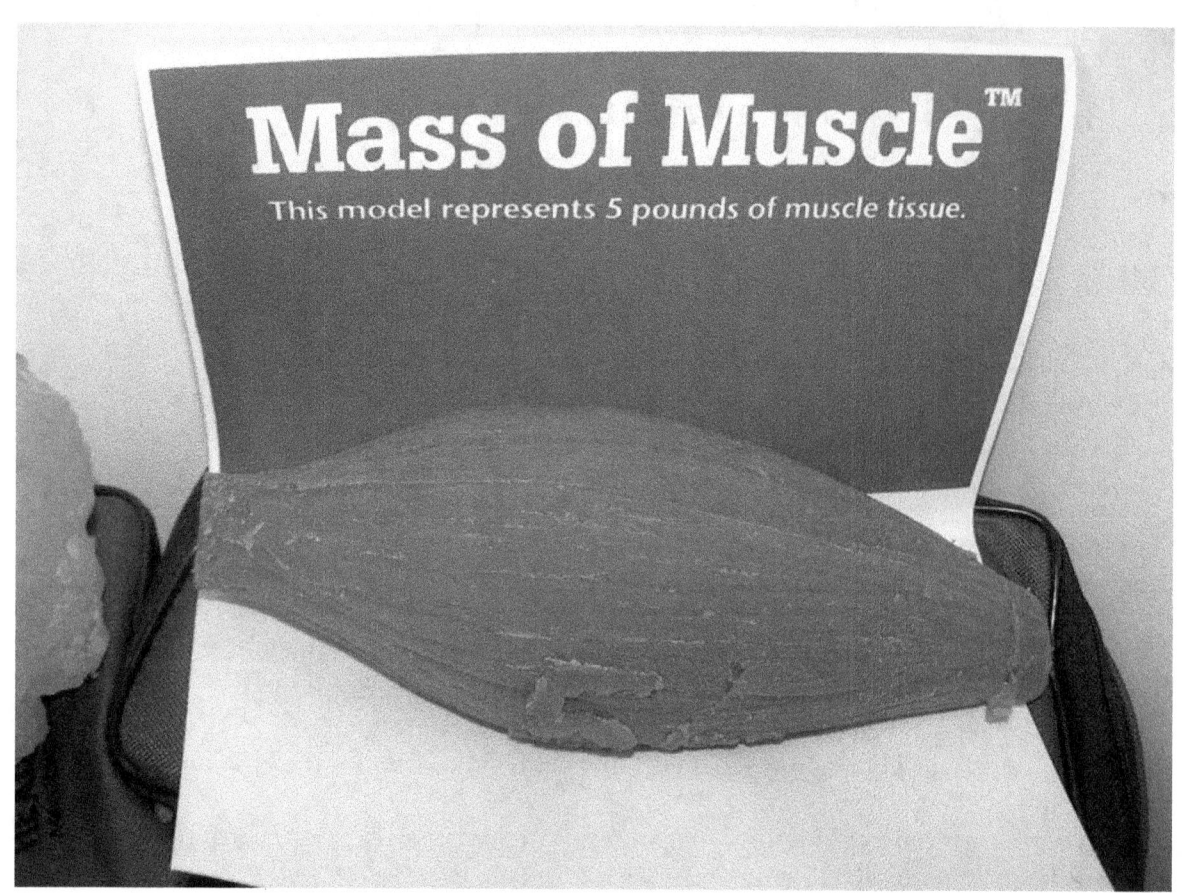

Here is shown a representation of 5 pounds of human muscle tissue

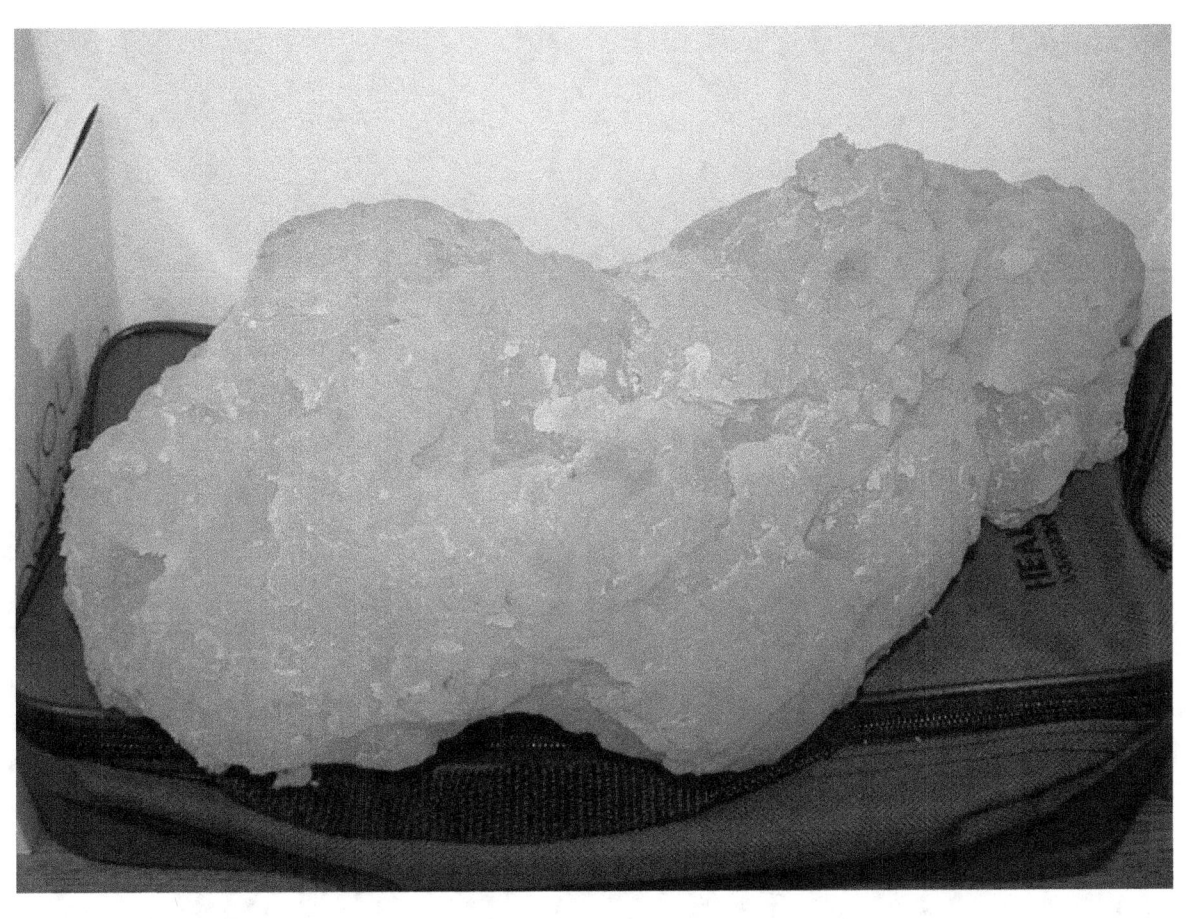

Here (above) we have 5 pounds of adipose (Fat) tissue

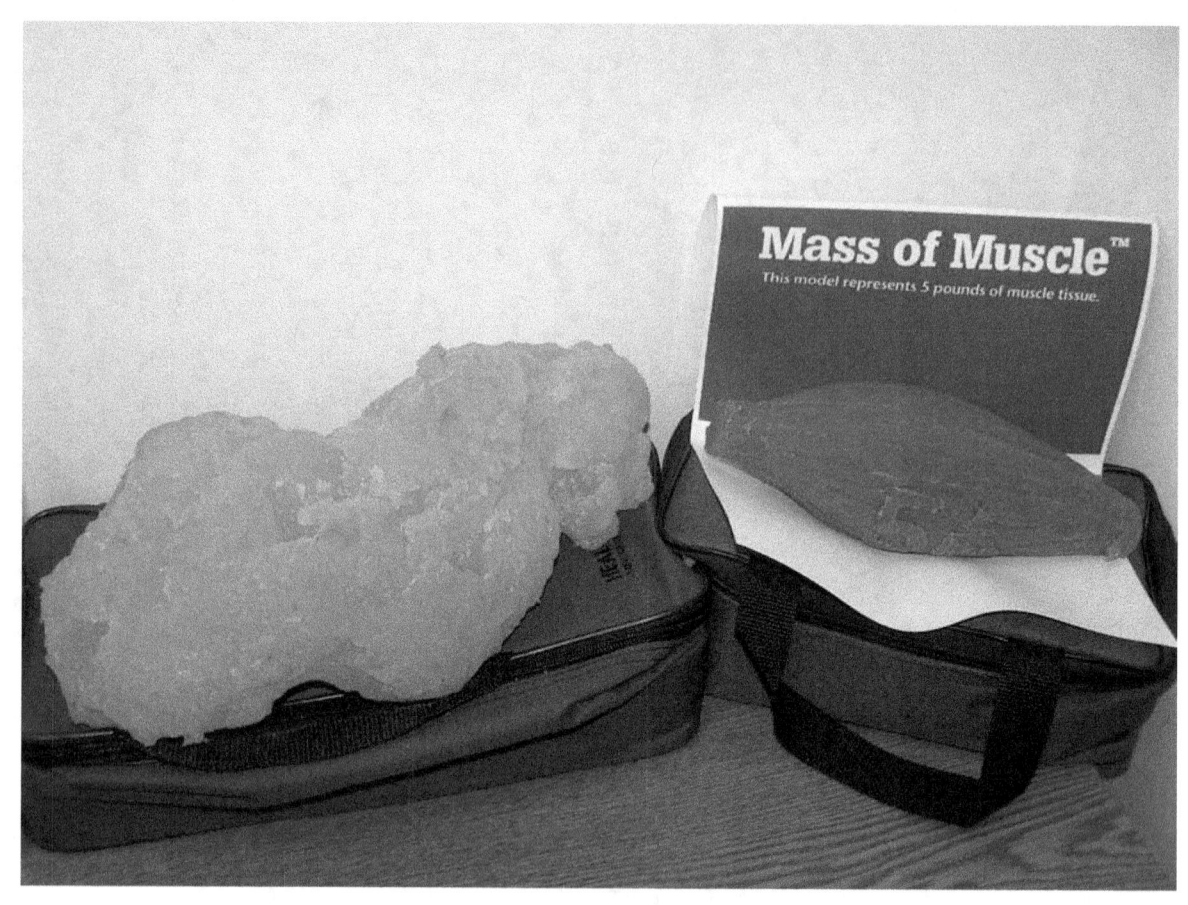

Above we see the 2 side by side, for a better comparison.

It is obvious from the photos above that Fat or adipose tissue takes up a lot more space for its mass than does muscle tissue.

Consider the difference in your body's appearance and overall health that would occur simply by losing 5-10 pounds of fat and gaining 5-10 pounds of muscle to replace it with. Of course, the net weight loss could end up being zero, but your fat/muscle ratio has dramatically changed for the better.

This is one reason that people who engage in the fitness lifestyle all the way around (Eating better, getting cardio work in and doing strength/muscle building work simultaneously) don't see big changes on the scale.

I advise them that the scale does not always tell the whole story, and that this should not discourage them.

Chapter 7

Supplements

As this is geared towards the older guys (middle aged and beyond), I will start with **supplements for the joints**. Many of us will need help in this area, especially if you've been pounding heavy weights for years as I have. **Glucosamine, MSM, Chondroitin, and Hyaluronic acid** are all beneficial, along with certain herbs. There are several formulas out there which contain all of the above. Different brands will have different "proprietary formulas" of herbs, minerals or vitamins to complement the standard 4 products mentioned above. I use one of these multi-products and it definitely helps, but does not eliminate joint issues altogether, at least in my case.

A friend of mine and former personal trainer recently told me about a supplement made by Natrol called **Cetylpure,** which is claimed to rebuild cartilage.

The active ingredient is **cetyl myristoleate**, which is a naturally occurring Fatty acid.

He claims it was implemental in recovering from knee injury in his past, and while I have no personal experience with this product, I have no reason to doubt my friend on this.

A **high potency multi-vitamin is a good idea**, especially if you don't have an optimal diet.

Beyond the above items, there is a long list of optional supplements you may want to consider. If you were to try every conceivable thing that might possibly be of help, you would probably go broke very quickly.

If you open the typical fitness or bodybuilding magazine these days, you will be bombarded by a myriad of ads for all kinds of "state of the art" supplements which make big promises. There's **more hype than substance to a lot of this stuff, but there are some products that seem to help at least some users.**

I am always looking for an edge and have tried lots of supplements in my day. The 2 most popular supplements used by a lot of lifters these days that I like are **Nitric Oxide and Creatine Monohydrate.**

There are many brands of both and some are better than others. Usually the old adage "you get what you pay for" holds true here also. Looking for the cheapest version of anything may bite you in the butt.

This is not always the case, however. Sometimes a lesser known brand that doesn't spend huge amounts of money on fancy packaging or advertising may be just as good as its flashier counterpart.

Try the cheaper brands to see if they might work just as well, sometimes you will be pleasantly surprised.

I have always gotten some benefits from any brand of creatine, but I prefer the straight creatine powder as opposed to the huge barrels that contain creatine and lots of sugar and other additives. **Using a high glycemic index juice like grape or apple juice is reported to facilitate uptake of the creatine by the muscles** and I prefer this over the commercial formulations.

The **downside to creatine** is that you will retain water (at least some of which is intra-muscular water, which makes them bigger), and potential muscle cramping. You must stay well hydrated to avoid the cramps. Your body actually gets creatine from dietary sources, such as red meat, but it's tough to get the amount you would get by simply adding a teaspoon per day (5 grams) of the powder.

Creatine is used by the body to manufacture ATP, the primary energy source for muscular contraction, so it stands to reason that supplementation would be helpful.

With that being said, **don't take more than recommended doses or stay on it indefinitely, as it puts an extra load on the kidneys, liver and digestive system.** It could possibly elevate blood pressure, so if you're hypertensive, you should probably leave it alone.

I use it during a heavy training period, for maybe 3 months tops, and then lay off it for a while. If you're trying to lose weight, avoid it like the plague!

Nitric Oxide or "NO2"

Nitric Oxide works by expanding the blood vessels, thus giving **a tremendous pump effect.** A side effect is that it can be helpful with ED, some report. Not a bad side effect!

Scientific studies have even suggested benefits for the heart, possibly even lowering high blood pressure. My experience has been that it helps me to recover more quickly and fully, which is a big help. Of course, this is "anecdotal evidence", and may not work the same for you personally.

Another popular supplement the days is the amino acid Glutamine.

When this is taken in isolated fashion, in doses of 5 or more grams after and/or before workouts, it is reported to help recovery considerably. I have been using it recently and it really does seem to help cut down on the **DOMS (delayed onset muscle soreness).**

Another issue faced by the older man is decreased testosterone production. Natural testosterone production varies greatly among normal individuals, by as much as a factor of ten or more.

There are numerous supplements that claim to boost this hormone, but the scientific field does not seem too convinced on many of these. Ginseng, horny goat weed, smilax, terrestris tribulus, wild yam, and yohimbe root are a few of the things reported to do this.

Androstenedione was very popular until largely banned, possibly being helped by the famous baseball player who was using it.

I have had mixed results with these things, but some seem to help at least in the short term. I actually got pretty decent results years back with something like Androstenedione, but the product was discontinued because of side effects, etc. Guess what, anything that works along these lines is almost definitely also going to have side effects, much as any drug would. More recently, I have tried horny goat weed and tribulus, and have not had outstanding results, though I can't say either is useless.

I suspect some of the proprietary formulas of herbal extracts may be more beneficial than just taking the straight herbs, but I have yet to try any of the newest formulations of these that are currently available. **Zinc supplements** can be good for the immune system as well as keeping the reproductive system running optimally, thus could be an aid to testosterone production. ZMA is a form of zinc that has been used to boost testosterone by some athletes, but I did not get much out of it when I tried it.

There are foods that are reported to enhance libido and/or performance, such as oysters.

The foods that are reported as such for the most part have one thing in common;

High levels of zinc, with also perhaps vitamin E and minerals like magnesium and potassium being relatively high.

Another popular substance is DHEA. Research is kind of a mixed bag on this from what I have read.

It may be beneficial to older men much more so than younger men, as the hormone decrease naturally in the body sometime after age 40- 50.

You may want to give it a try if you are in this age bracket or beyond.

Even supplementing Garlic has been reported to be helpful in this area, not just for helping with bringing down cholesterol levels and helping with heart issues.

Testosterone production is boosted just by working out hard. High intensity weight training on the basic compound exercises fits the bill. Overdoing cardio, not getting enough rest or proper nutrition will have a negative effect on testosterone production, and this is a primary reason why novices to intermediate trainees fail to make gains by emulating programs of more advanced lifters that are getting help from steroids.

I could go on about this topic, but I'll leave it at that for now.

Chapter 8

Flexibility

This is another **vital topic for the mature lifter.** It's important for everyone, but especially for the older enthusiast. **Stretching is an absolute must**, as is a good warm-up, before any heavy lifting or other strenuous activity is attempted.

Let me clarify; warm-up before lifting, but do not stretch before warm-up. **Never try to stretch a cold muscle.** Muscles are more "brittle" when they are cold, and much more prone to injury. This also means lifting in a cold environment can be dangerous. I like to use "**active recovery**". This means on my off days, I do my stretching and trunk exercises.

Stretching during or after a workout is fine, if you have the time. There are various types of stretching; static, ballistic, pnf, etc.

I do not suggest ballistic stretching, especially for a novice trainee. This involves a sudden "jolt" into the stretch position. I consider this dangerous, especially from a cold start. Static stretching is just holding a stretched position, like touching toes for a certain period of time. These are O.K, but not **the best, in my opinion. PNF is "proprioreceptive neuromuscular facilitation"** Yes, that is quite a mouthful, huh?

It is kind of a combination of static stretching and isometric contractions, to simplify it.

In other words, one starts out with a mildly stretched position, and exerts some force against a partner or inanimate object (I.E. a wall or doorway) at this position, for about 5 seconds. Then, you relax momentarily, and follow with a slightly deeper stretch position, hold/push there, continue process until stretch becomes uncomfortable. This enables a deeper stretch while promoting strength at the same time. I use this and find it to be the best form of stretching I've used.

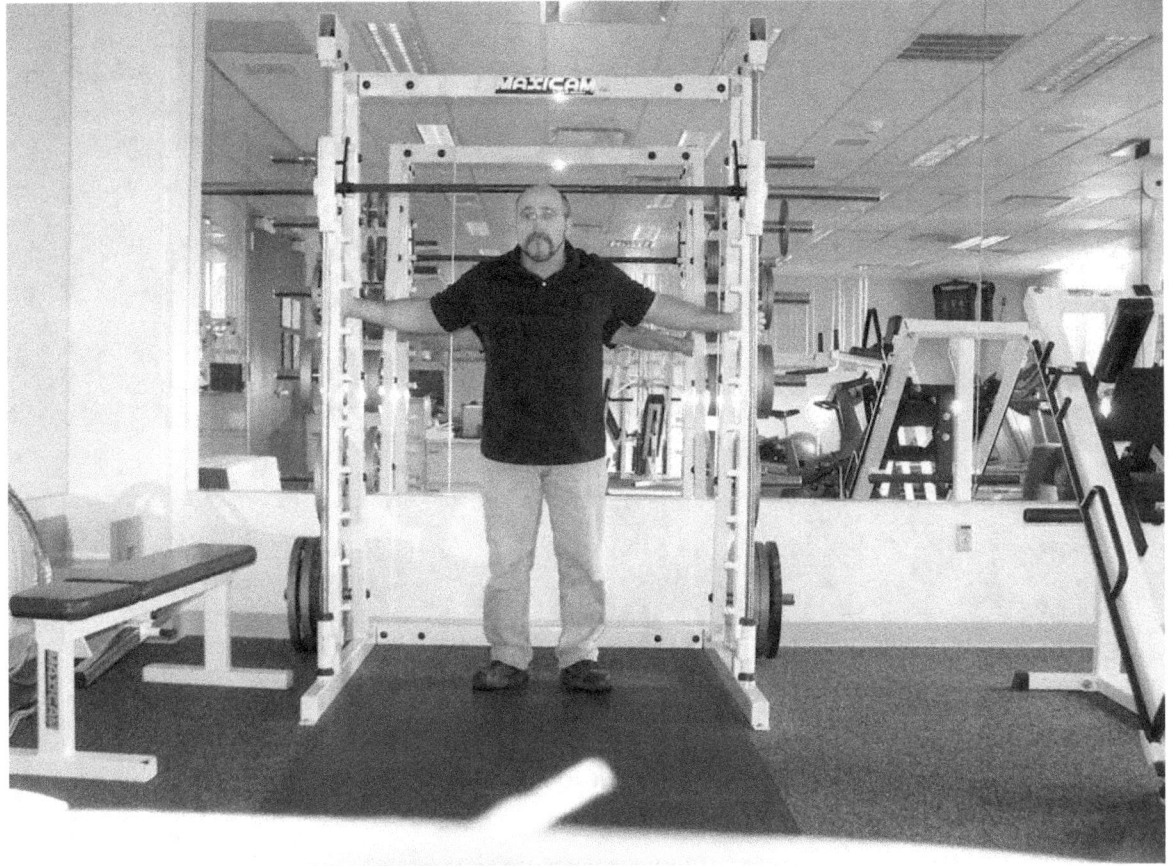

Here is an example of using a stationary object to do assisted PNF stretching.

Push against the uprights from a mildly stretched position, and hold for 5 seconds. Relax and then go into a slightly deeper stretch, push and hold for 5 seconds again.

Continue this several times until you have reached as deep a stretch as you can comfortably manage

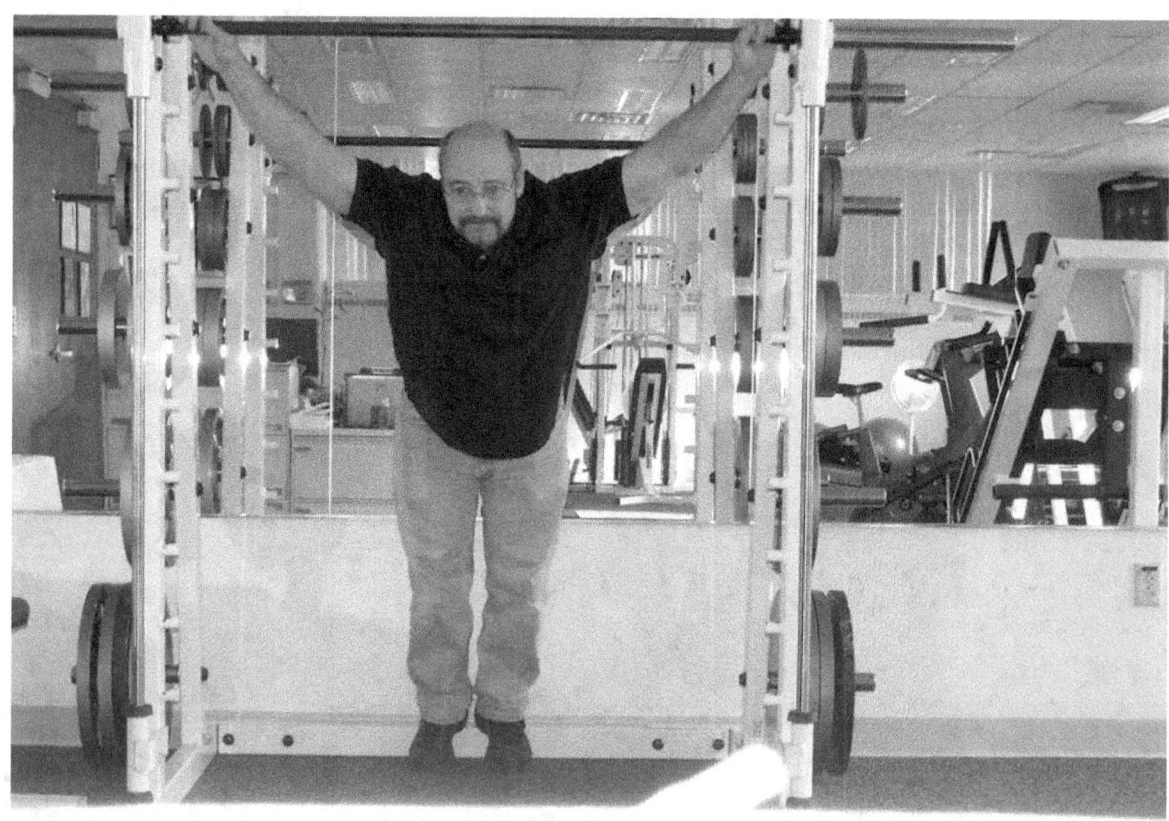

In the above photo, I am leaning forward while holding and pushing down against the fixed bar. This stretches the lats and delts. Perform in the same fashion as that shown above on pec stretch.

☺

In the photo below is shown a stretch for the quadriceps (front leg). As you hold the leg with opposite hand, push against the resistance of the hand with the leg muscles, and again hold that position for 5 seconds. Pull the leg to a deeper stretch position; hold/push for another 5 seconds. Continue process until deepest stretch possible is obtained.

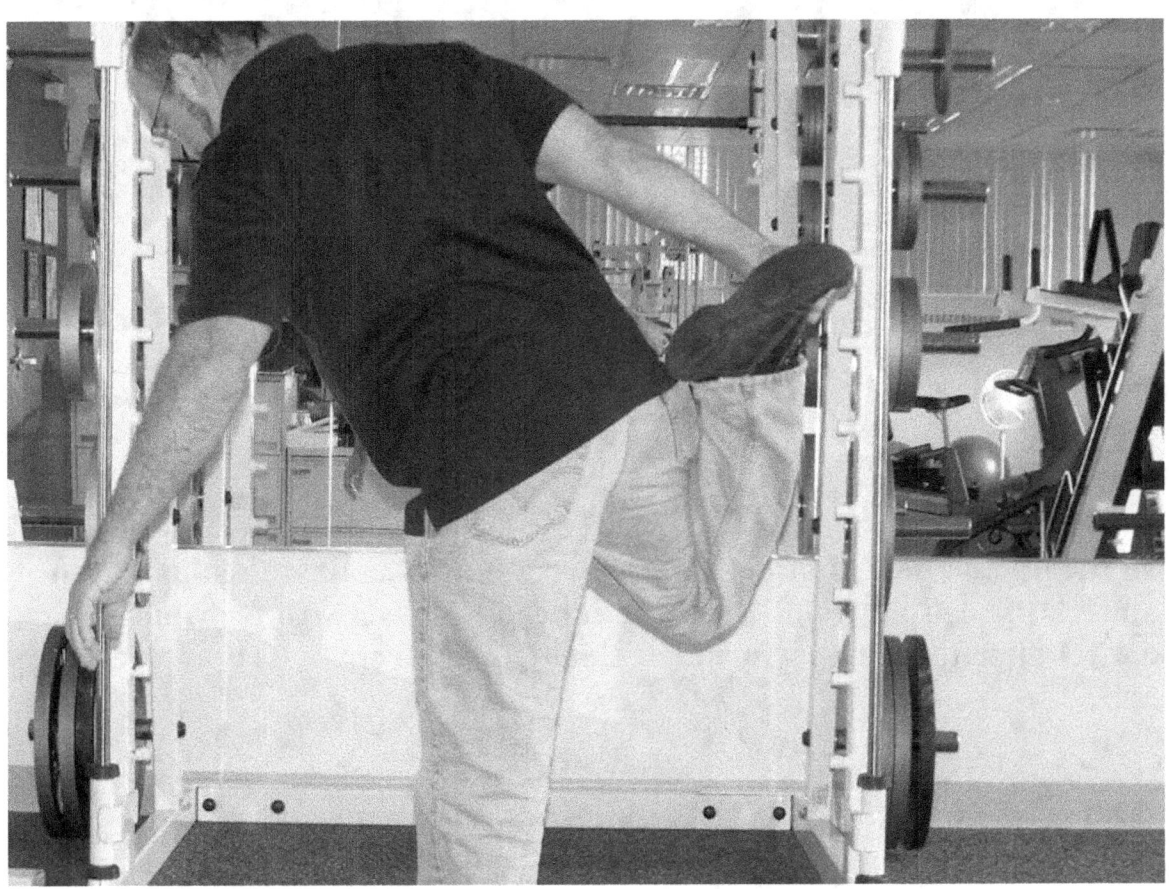

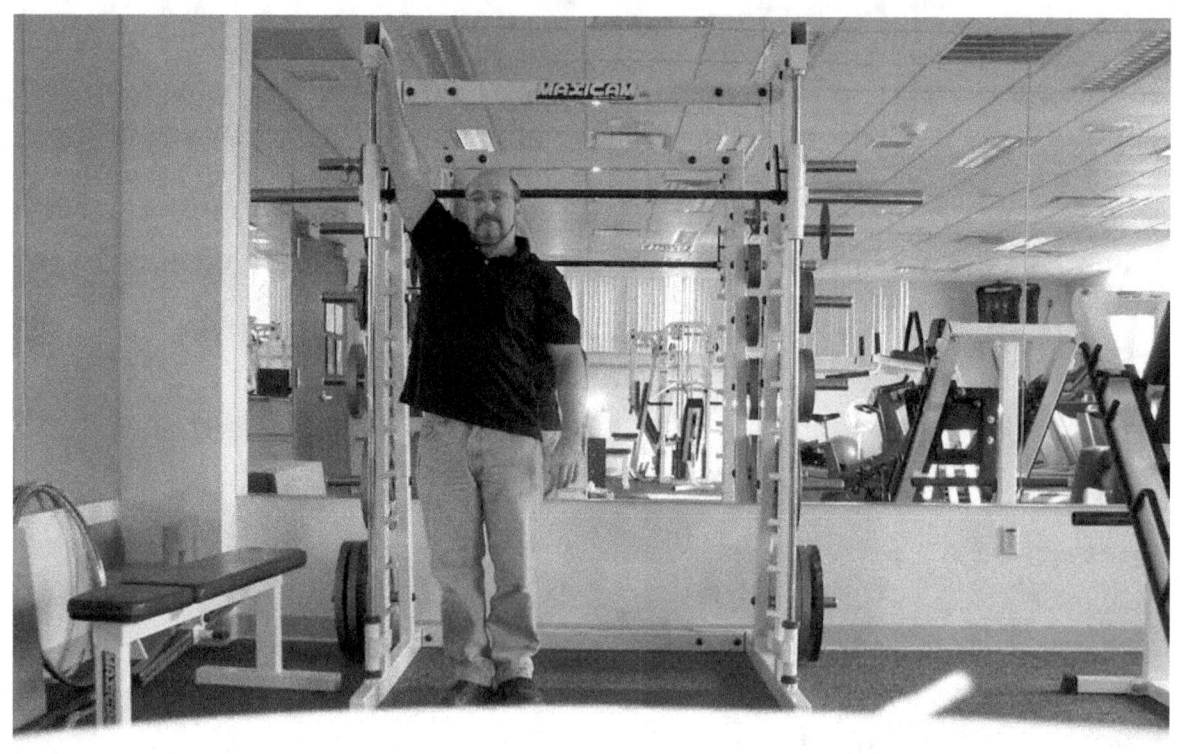

In the photo above, I am pushing my right arm against the upright to stretch the deltoid, using the same concept as described previously. Switch to left side to perform left side deltoid stretch.

In the photo below, I am performing a stretch for the low back using similar technique to that described above. I am pushing against my lower legs, while trying to push my upper body to the upright position with my lower back strength (you have to concentrate on this). After the initial push/hold, I would descend lower and push again

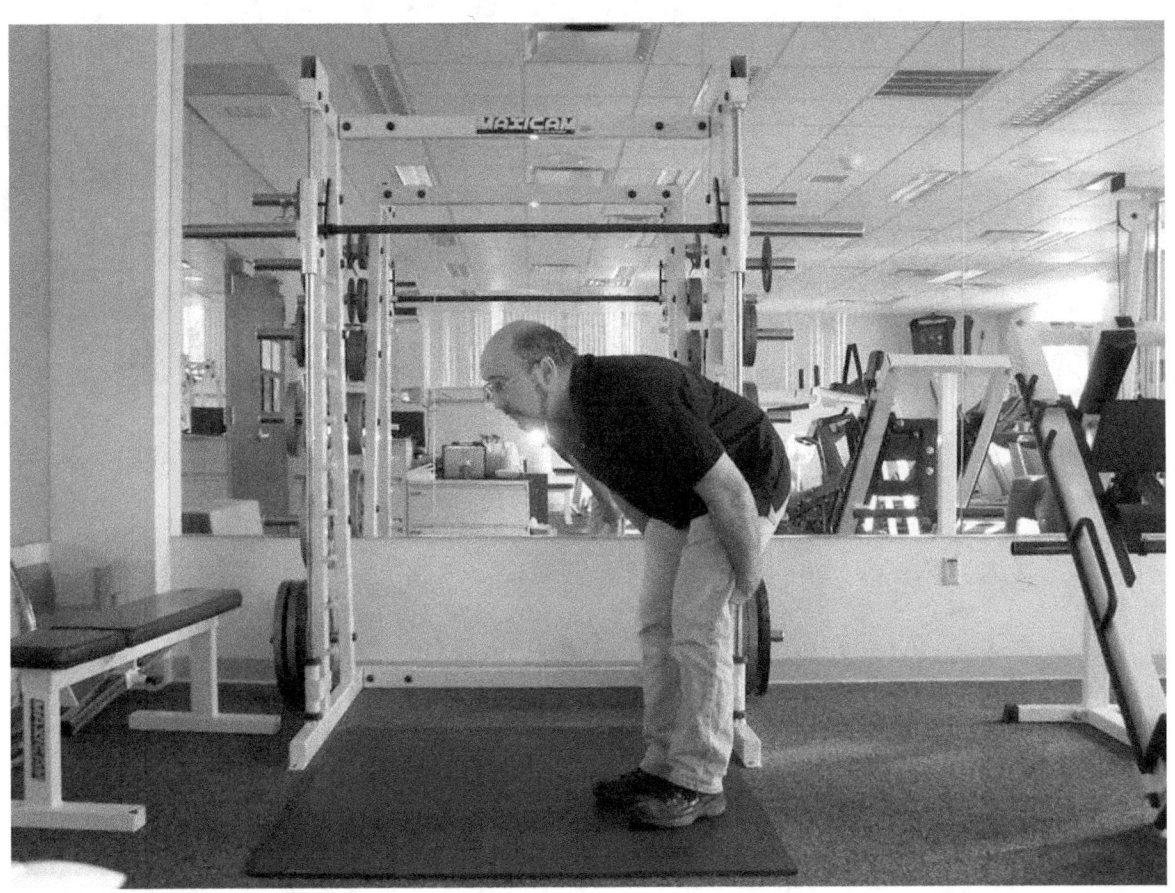

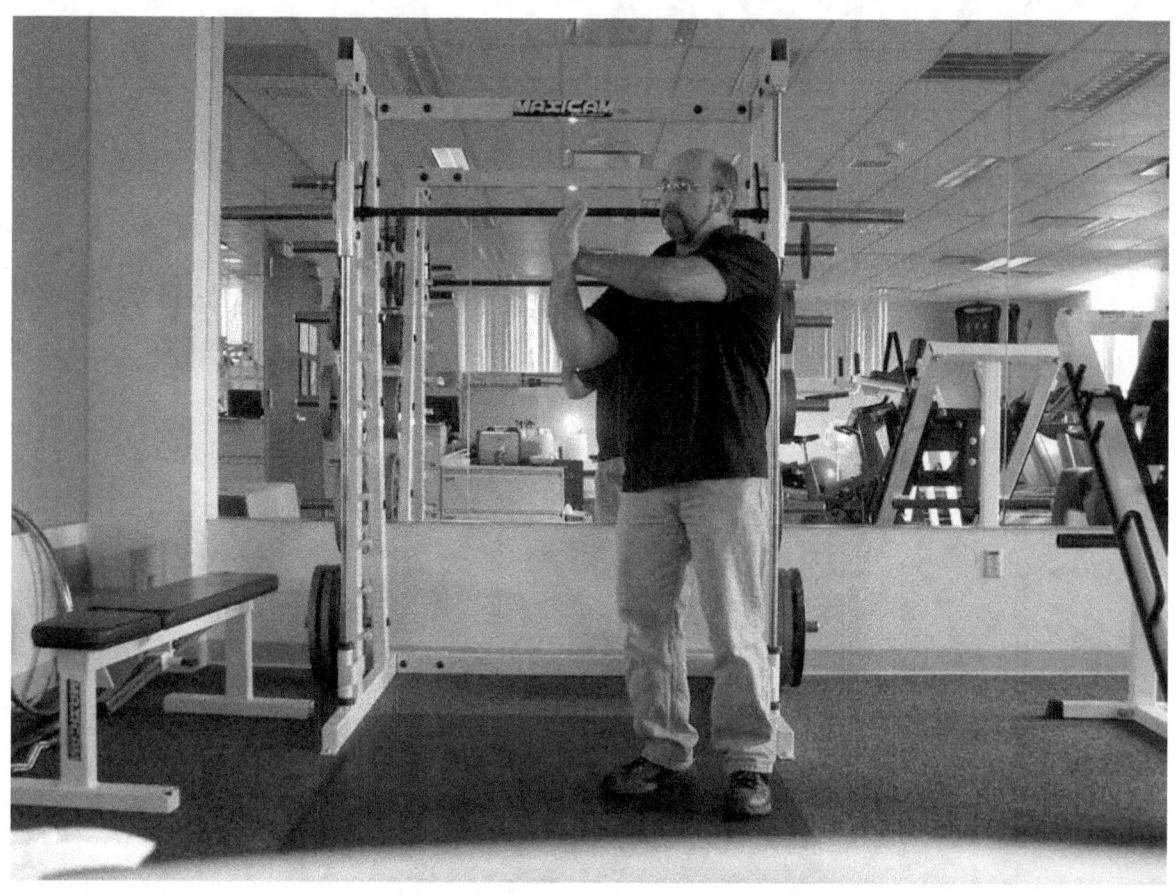

In the above demonstration, I am stretching the right triceps by pushing against the left arm from a mildly stretched position. Follow the procedures as outlined above.

Below, I am stretching the forearm by holding it in a stretched (twisted) position while performing the push/hold technique.

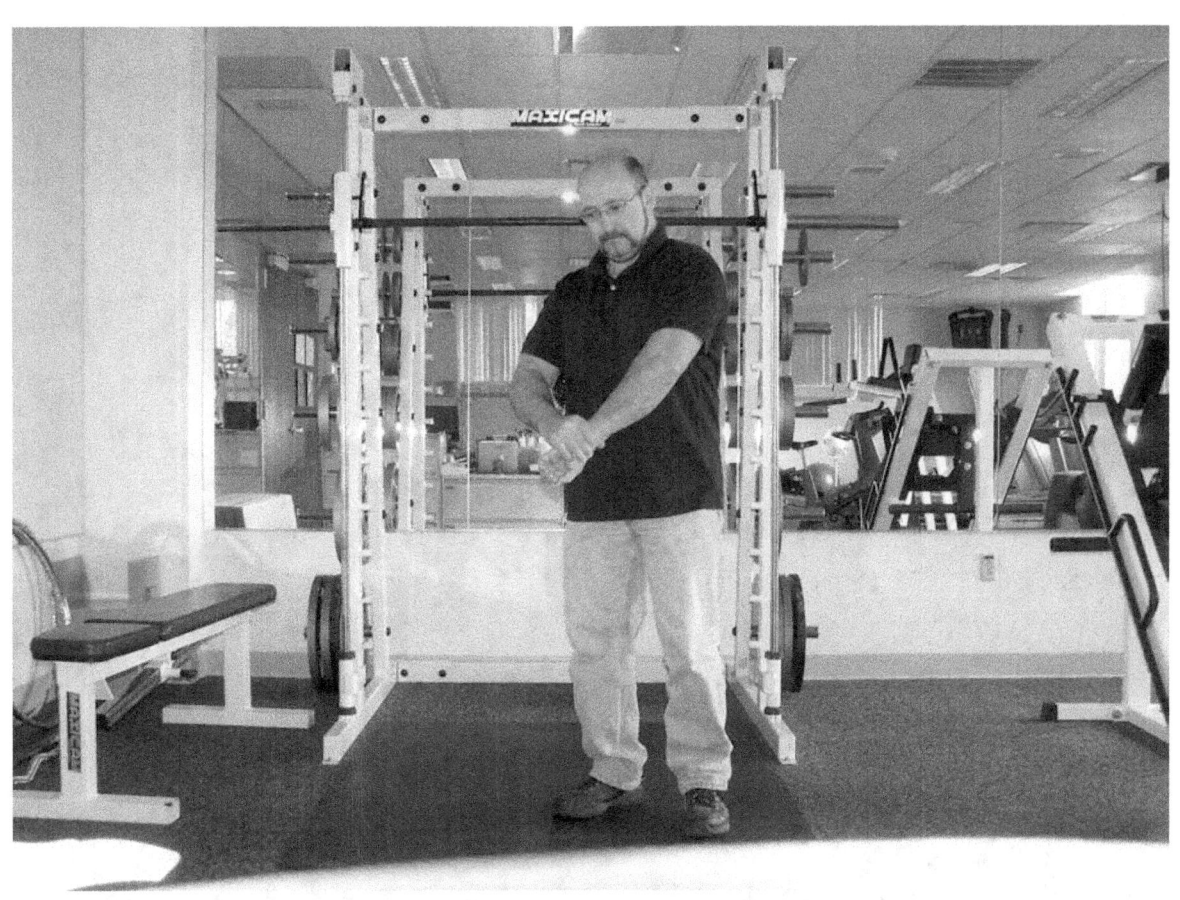

Below is a stretch for the biceps muscle in same format.

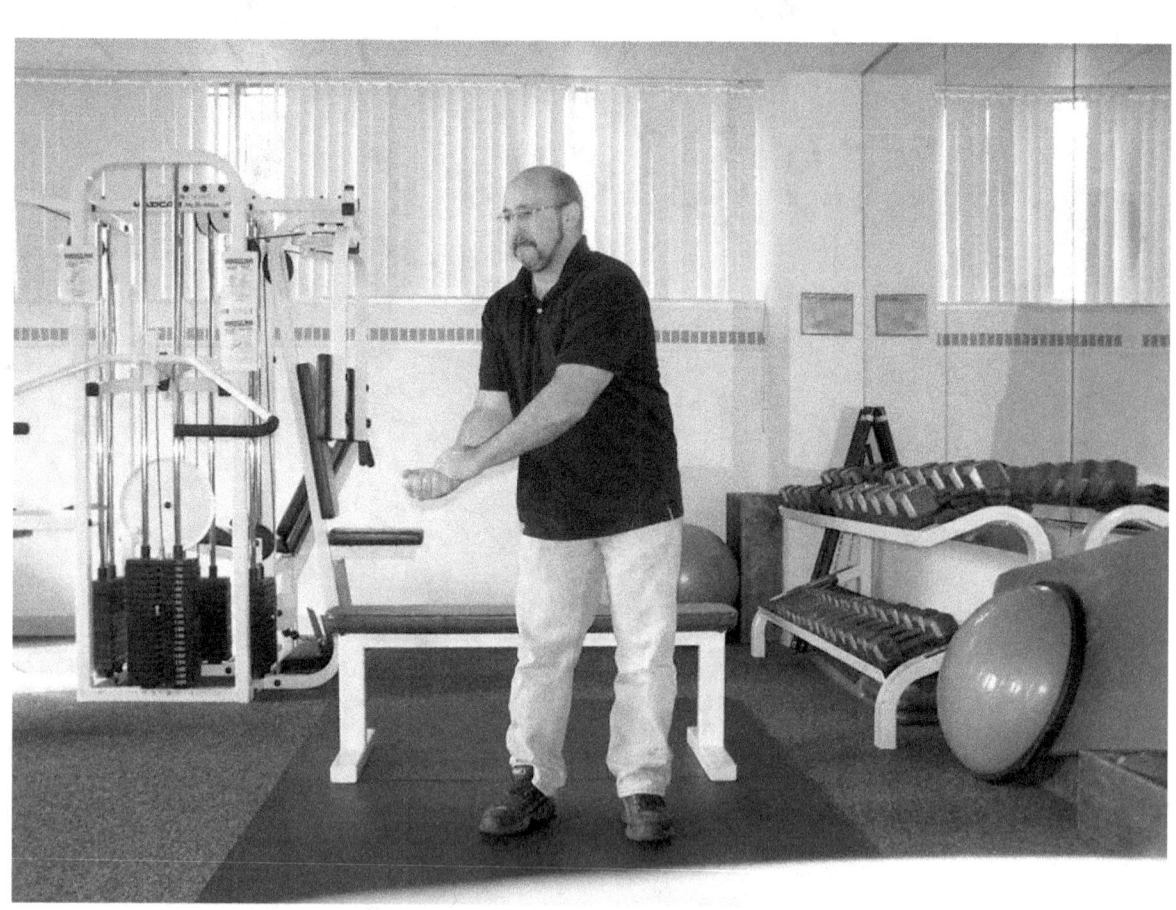

Below is shown a hamstring stretch using a barbell bar as fixed resistance point.

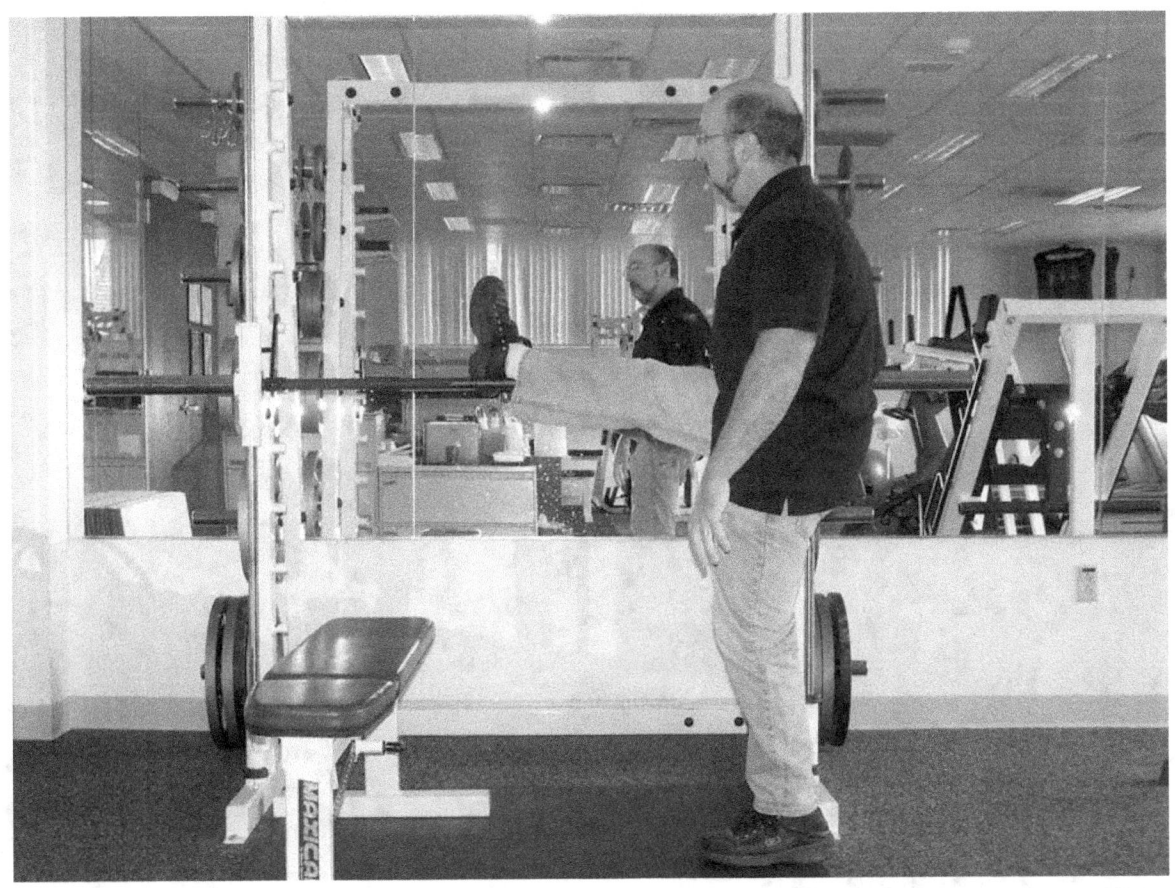

In the picture below, I am doing a "static" stretch for the groin/inner thigh. I will try to hold position for a few seconds, then go to a deeper stretch. I will continue until full stretch is reached, then switch sides and continue in the same fashion.

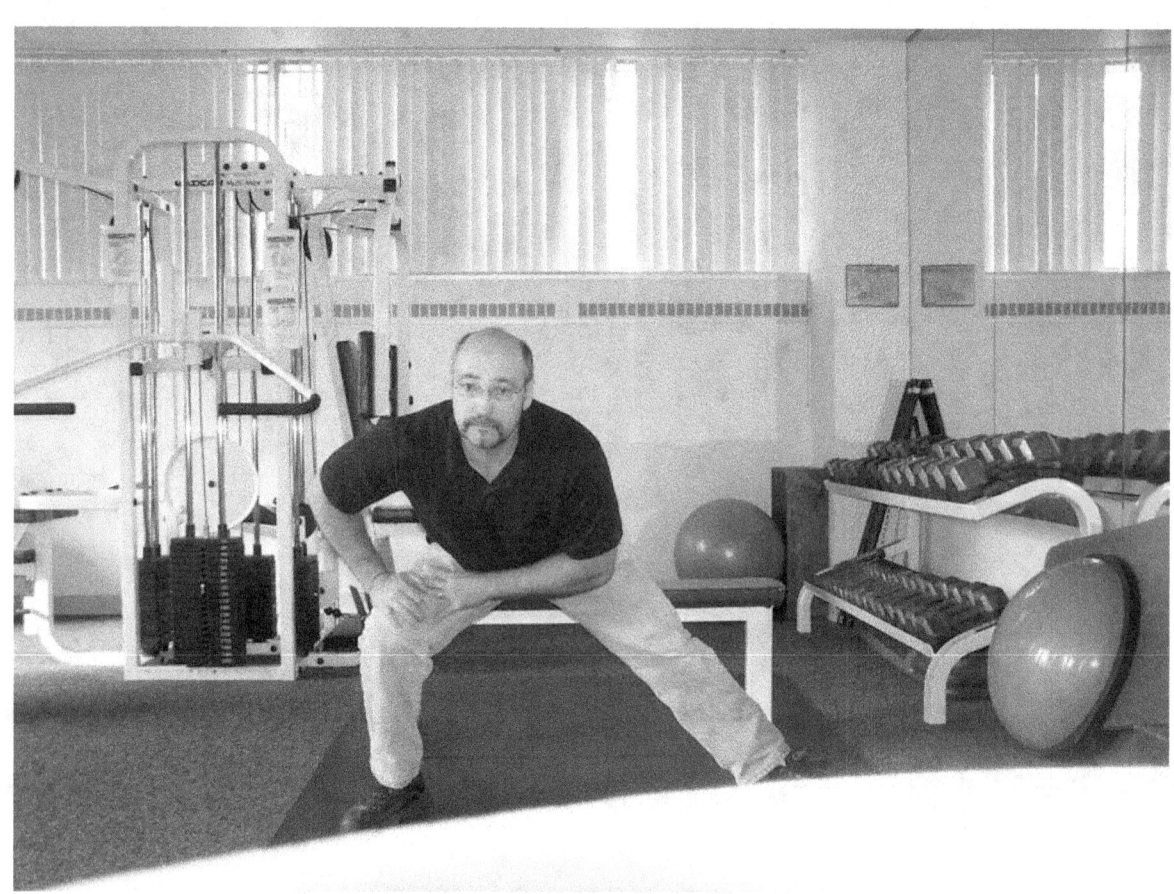

Below you see the "Wall Crawl". Bending backwards, I try to gradually get my hands lower on the wall while stretching the back further. This is a challenging stretch!

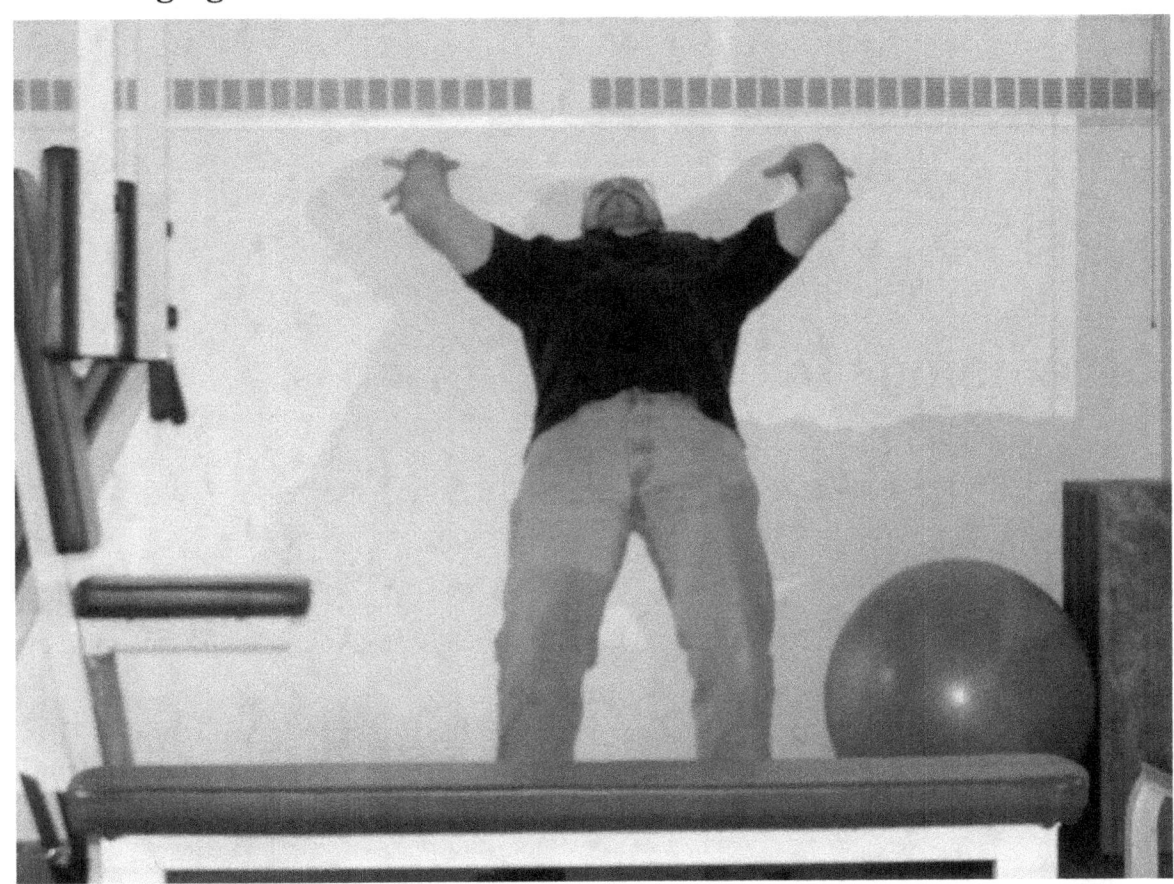

There are other ways of getting more flexible. **Yoga, Tai Chi, Pilates, and similar forms** may help in this regard. Doing some calisthenics can help keep you get limber, and can be a good warm-up for weight training.

For those with limited time, a whole routine could be made up of **calisthenics**, actually.

A more flexible muscle is a stronger muscle and a healthier muscle. Neglecting this area would be a huge mistake. I have in the past gone that route and suffered from the results; Torn and strained muscles, lost training time, etc. It was just too easy to forget or let slide, but I make sure these days to get it in somehow. For me, using off days and just dedicating about 20 minutes to a stretching/ trunk session seems to work well. I swear by it.

Chapter 9

Other things to consider

There are other things to think about, and they don't really fit into a specific category, but are worthy of mentioning.

Muscle rubs like mineral ice, icy-hot, tiger-balm and the like can be useful for us old timers. When I'm training for a big lift, or competition I'll use it before working out to help in the warming process. You might find it helpful, but don't use it for every workout.

Breathing Techniques are a very important but often overlooked area. Breathing through the nose is superior to mouth breathing, primarily because there's more filtering going on. Also, one should practice breathing as deeply as possible with every breath. I'm not talking about breathing while working out, but everyday normal breathing.

Yoga practitioners are big on this, and it is the first lesson of the form usually. We get our "life force" from oxygen, so it stands to reason that taking in as much as we can, with each breath will be helpful.

Concentrate on filling the abdomen with air first, then gradually expanding the rib cage, then bringing air all the way up into the top of the lungs. It takes practice, and it should not be a 3 or 4 part breath, but should be one fluid movement eventually. **This slows the resting heart rate, relaxes the entire body, and just generally invigorates.** Read some yoga or Tai-chi manuals about breathing for a better, more detailed explanation of this.

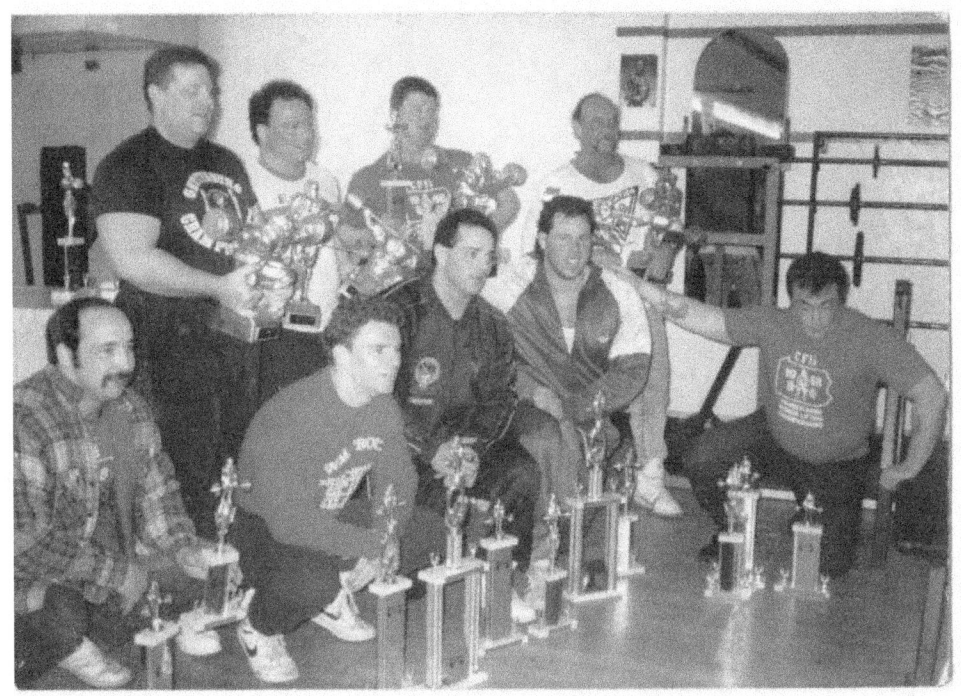

Competing

Competition, while not for everybody, **can be a fun and exciting way to motivate you to train harder and/ or more consistently**. These days, there are many outlets for those who are competitive in spirit. In the strength arena, there are power lifting meets consisting of one or all three of the conventional big three; bench, squat or deadlift In addition, many now offer curling, repetition bench press and other "odd-lifts" as part of the overall competition. Strongman contests and arm wrestling are also pretty popular.

 If you are into running and other endurance sports, 5k races, triathlons, marathons and other such competitions are available widely.

Chapter10

The Mental aspect

If] you faint in the day of adversity, your strength *[is]* small.Prov24:10

This chapter could really be a book by itself. **The mind is so important in any physical endeavor, it can not be overstated. If you don't think positively, your results are hardly going to be positive.**

If you can not visualize yourself performing well, you will not perform well. It is just that simple.

This is especially true for those competing in sports that require a short term, all out effort, like doing a 1 rep max in a power lifting contest.

One phenomenon that strongly supports the mind-body link is **the placebo effect**, which is what causes people taking a pill that they are told contains a drug or medicine that will help them do something or alleviate something, to actually get the desired effect, despite the fact that the pill contains no active ingredient.

In just about every double blind drug efficacy study ever done, some people claim to get the drugs desired results from taking a sugar pill.

This same phenomenon is what helps keep a lot of supplement and diet aid companies in business.

Think about it! If you convince someone that the pill you are giving them will help them lose weight (for example), a certain percentage of these folks will lose weight, even if the pill is nothing but talcum powder. Now, you use these folks to do testimonials. Anecdotal evidence can be obtained to support almost anything you want it to support.

In my early days of lifting with buddies in my parent's garage, I learned a nice trick to help friends go beyond their sticking points. I would add just a little more weight on the bar than my pal was expecting, without his knowledge. This often resulted in the lifter doing a new personal record, thinking he was just doing the same old same old routine.

Martial artists and Yoga practitioners, among others **understand the importance of the total focus that is needed to overcome physical obstacles**. "Chi" is the force they refer to.

Hypnotism, whether self-imposed or brought on by a hypno-therapist, is really nothing but extreme, concentrated focus. Another term for this is **"auto-suggestion"**

A word for the Christian about hypnosis here; it has often been associated with occultism and therefore shunned by Christians. There are those that say the step of "clearing the mind" is something that could open one up to evil, even demonic powers. To be sure, hypnosis could be used by someone with evil intentions.

I think that **getting in a very relaxed frame of mind, and then feeding your mind some positive suggestions,** I.E, You are getting stronger every day, or I can't wait for my next workout, and things along these lines can only be beneficial. Also, negative reinforcement, such as; cigarettes are filthy and disgusting, I can't stand them! Or, donuts and candy are my worst enemy, etc, etc, can also be helpful.

I get motivated by people telling me I can't do something. The best way to get me to achieve something is to tell me it is impossible, or that I'm an idiot to even think I could do such a thing. My training partners and I used this method on each other sometimes. I'd say something like "my grandma could do reps with that weight, you punk", perhaps followed by a crisp slap in the face. Sounds harsh, maybe a little weird, but it can work. Just don't try it on a stranger, that's all!

Visualization is a strong and well used technique. If you can visualize yourself doing an extra rep, or maxxing out with a few pounds more than your old personal best, you will have a much improved chance of actually doing it. If you think, this is too heavy, or I can't do that many reps, you've already defeated yourself, and your body will simply follow through on that negativity.

Motivation is something that everyone knows is vital in performing at top levels in any arena, yet it is not always clear where we can derive it from.
For some, a picture of themselves in very poor condition may be posted up on the refrigerator. This would be a form of "negative reinforcement"
For others, having life-sized posters or pictures of their favorite lifters or bodybuilders on the walls of their training area can help them to get motivated by imagining themselves in similar condition.
Imagining oneself in even seemingly ridiculous, exaggerated form, with 25 inch biceps and a 70 inch chest can be highly inspiring during an intense workout.

In my second book, "**Forgotten Secrets of the Old time Strongmen**", I mention what the great Eugene Sandow said about training intensity.

He said that doing one set of a particular exercise with absolute 100% focus was worth 10 sets done in a hap-hazard or "going through the motions" style.

Many other impressive men from the past held similar ideas, and I firmly believe in this concept myself.

I would even tell you that one of the reasons that steroids or artificial testosterone works like it does is because of the **aggressive attitude** it instills.

To be sure, there are things going on physiologically there that cause muscle & strength gain to result from your hard workouts, but you have to perform those gut wrenching workouts to get the results.

Steroids would be of little benefit to someone who didn't put the hard work in. If you can get yourself in a similar state of mind without the steroids, I think you have won at least half the battle.

Arnold spoke of lifting with "**Joy and Fierceness**" and while this may sound odd to some folks, I think he was right on the mark.

Of course, I am speaking of heavy strength training as opposed to a cardio or running workout for distance when I mention this.

Long endurance or cardio work also requires motivation and mental toughness of a different sort.

You might imagine yourself flying through the air while you are running, or something like this.

Think of breathing in strength, health & vigor with every burning inhalation of fresh oxygen, and expelling toxins and all things negative from your body on every exhalation.

Imagine yourself being able to run effortlessly up and down hills for miles and miles.

Think about how strong your lungs, heart and circulatory system are becoming as you run.

Think about the calories of fat you are melting off your body.

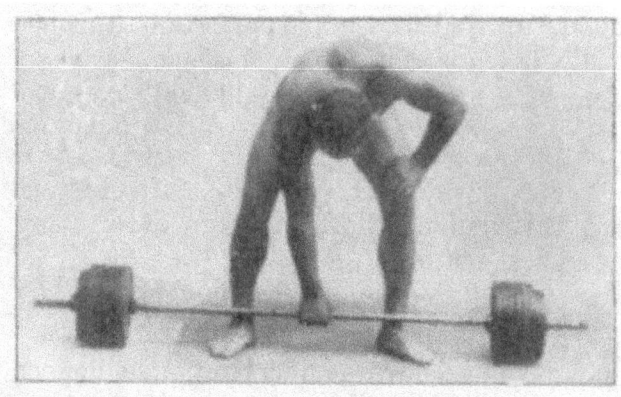

FIRST POSITION FOR BAR-BELL SNATCH OR FOR
ONE-HANDED JERK (CONTINENTAL STYLE).

Chapter 11

Developing your program

Now it is time to get down to the nitty- gritty. Let's build your personalized program.

I will present a sort of Ala carte menu of exercises from which you can choose. **Try to choose the ones you will enjoy,** or at least can tolerate most.

Free Weight Exercises	Muscles trained
Barbell bench press	Chest, shoulders, triceps
Barbell incline bench press	Upper chest, shoulders, and triceps
Squat	Legs, hips, and lower back
Deadlift	Lower back, hips, legs

Barbell bent over row	Upper back, biceps, low back
Barbell bicep Curl	Biceps, brachialis
Lying triceps extension (a.k.a head knockers)	Triceps
Seated military press	shoulders, triceps
Seated behind neck press	shoulders, trapezius
Dumbbell lateral raise	Shoulders (mid part)
Dumbbell pullover	Chest, upper back, triceps
Dumbbell fly	chest, shoulders
Barbell or dumbbell shrugs	Traps (rear upper back)
Wrist curl	forearms
Calf raises	calves
Lunges	legs

Bodyweight Exercises

Pushup	chest, shoulders, triceps
Chin-up	upper back, biceps
Dip between chairs	triceps, shoulders, and chest
Squat or Deep knee bend	legs, low back, hips
Squat-thrust	Legs, back, hips

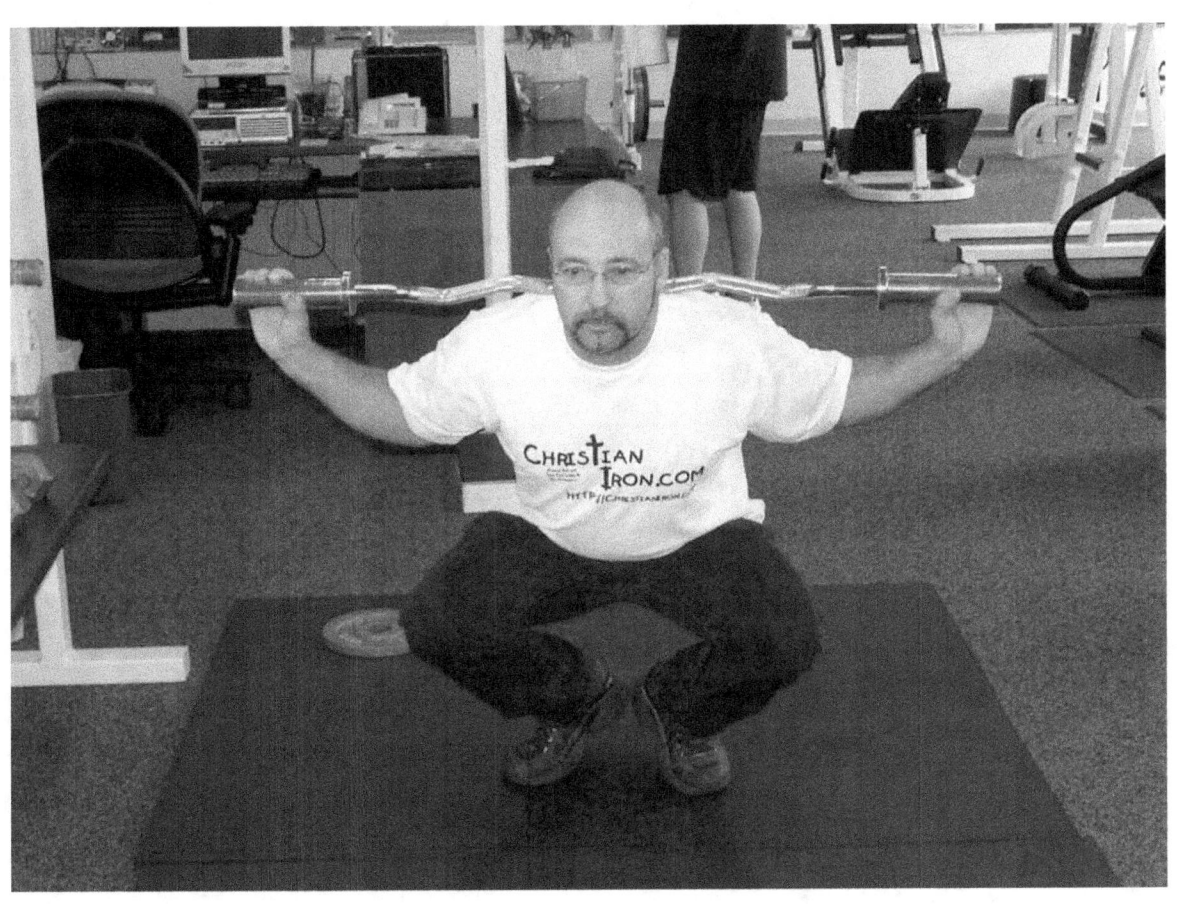

Above is shown the "Hindu Squat"
This can be done with no weight, just an empty bar as shown,
or a loaded barbell for a real challenge.
Note that the heals are raised and touching each other
throughout the movement.

Crunch	abdominals
Sit-up	abdominals
Leg lifts or raises	abdominals
Hand stand pushup (advanced level)	shoulders
Triceps, behind back dip	triceps, shoulders
Jumping jack	legs, minor upper body, cardio
Rope climbing	general upper body
Monkey bar hand walks	general upper body
Lunges	legs
Lying back extension	back
Simulated bike movement on back	legs, mild cardio

Cardio

Walking   jogging   running   treadmill   biking   swimming

Jumping rope   jumping on trampoline   run in place   elliptical machine

*Jumping jacks   * squat thrusts   stair climbing   use rowing machine

*mountain climbers   * Sled work, *playground drills *Tire flipping

Use bicycle/rowing combo type machine (cardio glide, etc) * Body only bike simulation

on back

Aerobic dance moves and related

-
- Note the items with asterisk above are higher intensity, callisthenic type moves, which should be kept to short duration.

Please note, **this is not an exhaustive list**, just some fundamental basic stuff. Keep in mind this is a "primer"

Notice the absence of machines that isolate specific muscles from the menu.

Frankly, I'm just not a huge believer in these, except as an adjunct to free weight training. Many commercial gyms strongly emphasize these moves for an entire routine or as part of a circuit training regimen. You could substitute leg presses for squats if you have knee or lower back issues, lat pull downs for rowing motions, or substitute a machine in any other move that you just find uncomfortable, but **I strongly prefer free weight moves to machines for most everything, especially for building strength, power and muscle mass**. I have never seen anyone develop a great deal of muscle mass by only using nautilus or similar machines.

Now, let's think back to the start of the book when we talked about making an honest time commitment evaluation.

Obviously, the more time you can give, the more different exercises you can do, or more time doing particular ones you're fond of you can spend

Also, **we have to consider our goals in making our choices from the menu**. If power, strength, and muscle size is what you are after, then I suggest sticking to things on the free weight menu primarily.

If you want toned muscles, perhaps a little strength gain but want to stay relatively lean, choices will tend to be in the bodyweight exercise section.

To lose weight, pick primarily from the cardio menu, with some strength building items from either or both of the other menus mixed in.

If time is at a premium, choose those items that fit into both categories like the calisthenics movements, with perhaps a little bodyweight or free weight training mixed in if time allows.

We want to keep things balanced, not over emphasizing any particular part of the body.

One way to do this is to do a lower body exercise for every upper body exercise, or a pushing exercise for every pulling exercise. An example is to do something like a bench press move (push) alternated with a rowing move (pull).

If you have a particularly weak body part or area, putting the emphasis there is OK until that are comes up to par, and I actually would suggest doing this.

Many folks do just the opposite, doing bench presses or curls every workout because they are good at it. Ever see somebody with huge arms and little else, or big upper body and stork like legs? Looks silly, eh? Also, it is not very functional in the real world.

Even if you have a lot of time on your hands, **don't spend hours in the gym**. Unless you are at a very advanced level, you can get good results from an hour or less of the strength phase of your program, and an hour of "slow burn" style of cardio is plenty.

More is not necessarily better, so don't get carried away.

Set short term goals for yourself, in line with your long term goals These goals should be achievable in a short time, relatively. This might mean losing 5 pounds in a month, adding 10 pounds to your bench repetition weight in a month, or something along these lines. When you reach a short term goal, set a new goal. If you fail to reach a goal, try to honestly evaluate why you failed

Did you stick to your plan? Is there a specific muscle area that seems to be lagging or holding you back? Did you at least make some progress? **If you made some progress but did not quite reach your goal, don't be too disappointed.**

You may need to adjust your goal to something more reasonable, or adjust your workout to meet the goal next time around. You need to experiment with different exercises, vary your routine, work on weak muscles a little harder.

If you feel tired or sore all the time, you may be overtraining, or are not getting enough sleep or good nutrition.

If you are putting in your cardio work and some strength training time, but not losing pounds, keep in mind you may be **gaining muscle and losing fat.** You should be using more weight in your workouts and feeling and looking better if that is the case.

Dieting alone or doing cardio and strength training alone is not nearly as effective as the combination of the two.

Chapter 12

Some Example Routines

Push-pull power, mass routine

Push
Monday

Bench Press
Warm up with very light weight for 20 reps or so, and then do 3 sets of 10-12 reps

Incline Press
Same scheme as above

Seated or standing military press
Same scheme

Lateral dumbbell raise
Same scheme

Finish with 6 sets Triceps work in same rep format, using
Lying triceps extensions, close grip bench press, kickbacks or bench dips (pick 2)

Do 100 reps abs

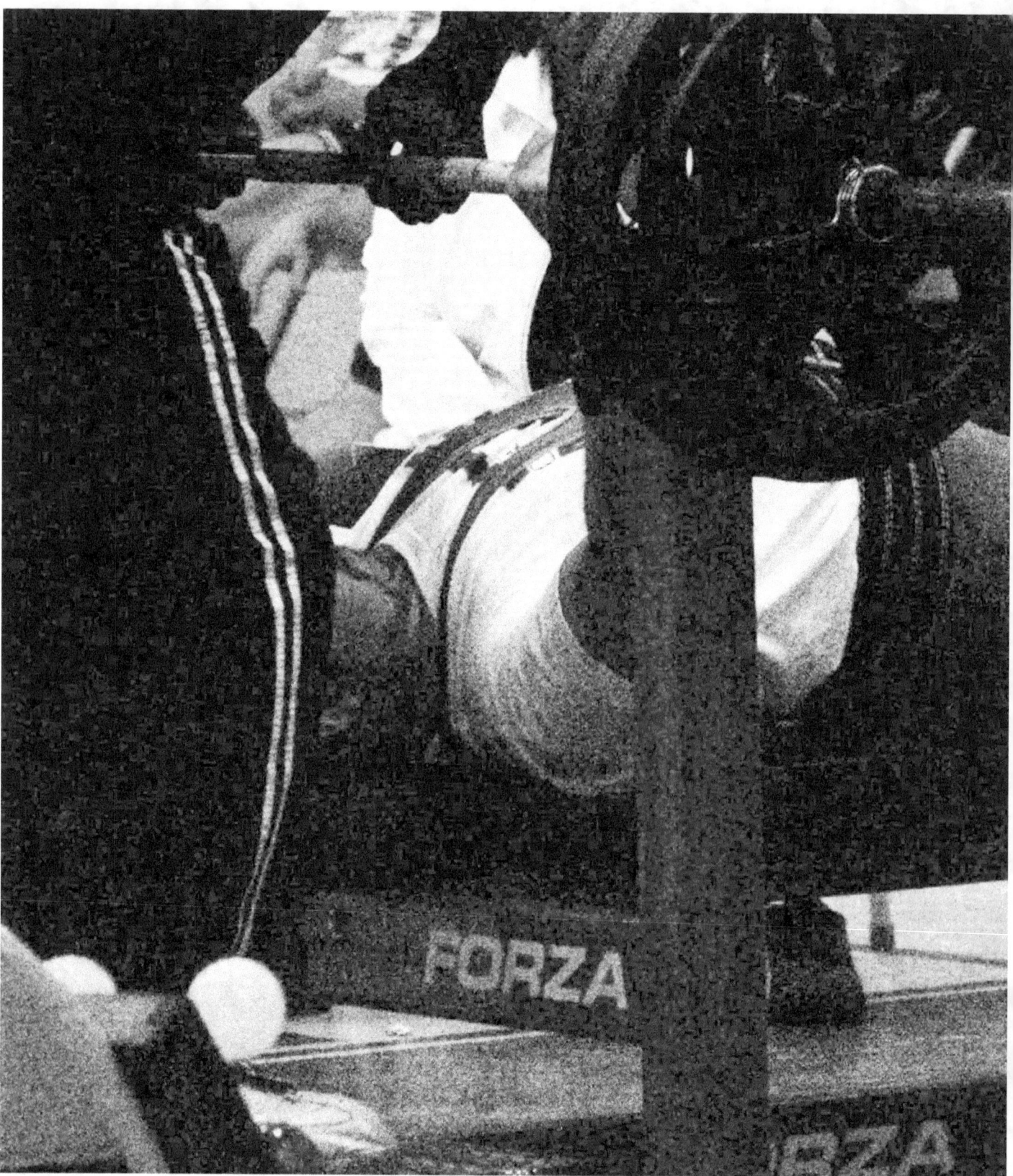

Above is the author performing a bench press at a competition

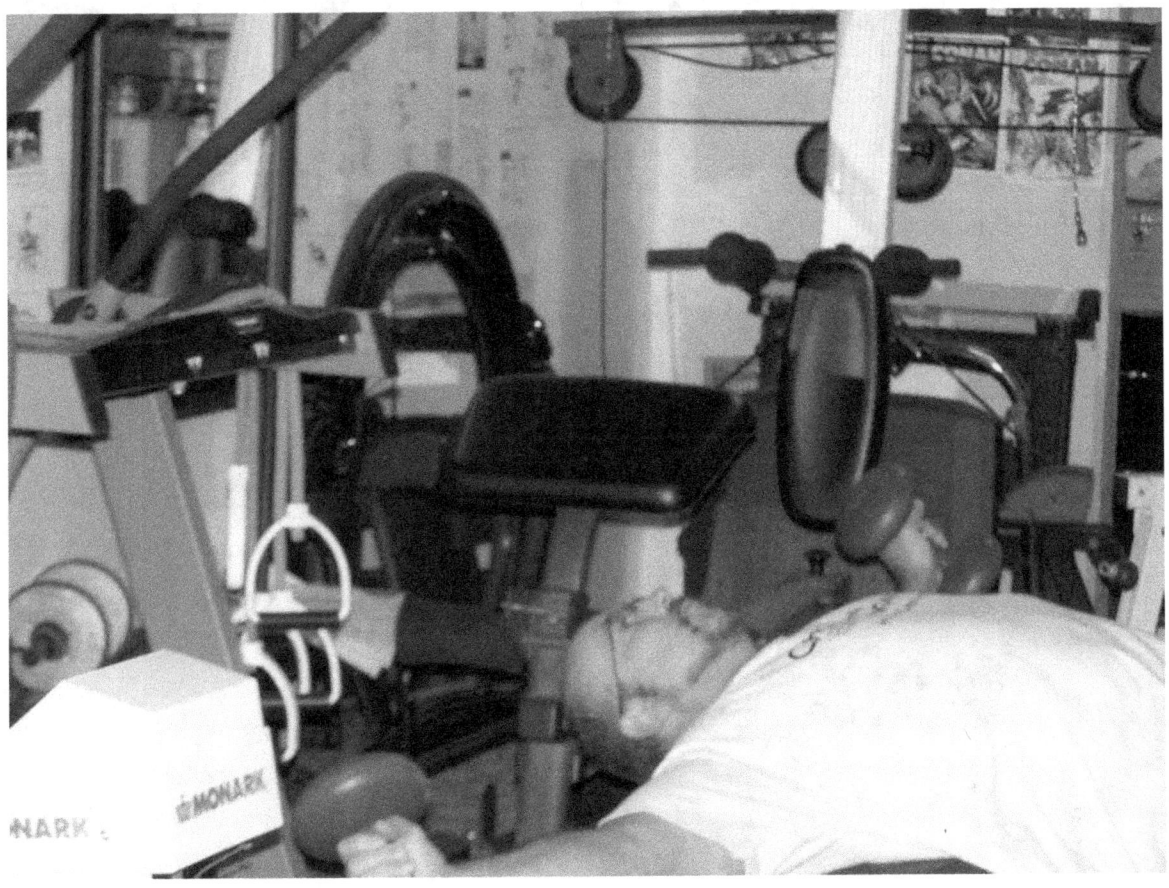

Here you see the bottom position of the dumbbell fly exercise

Below is the top of the fly exercise. This is the straight armed version of the fly.

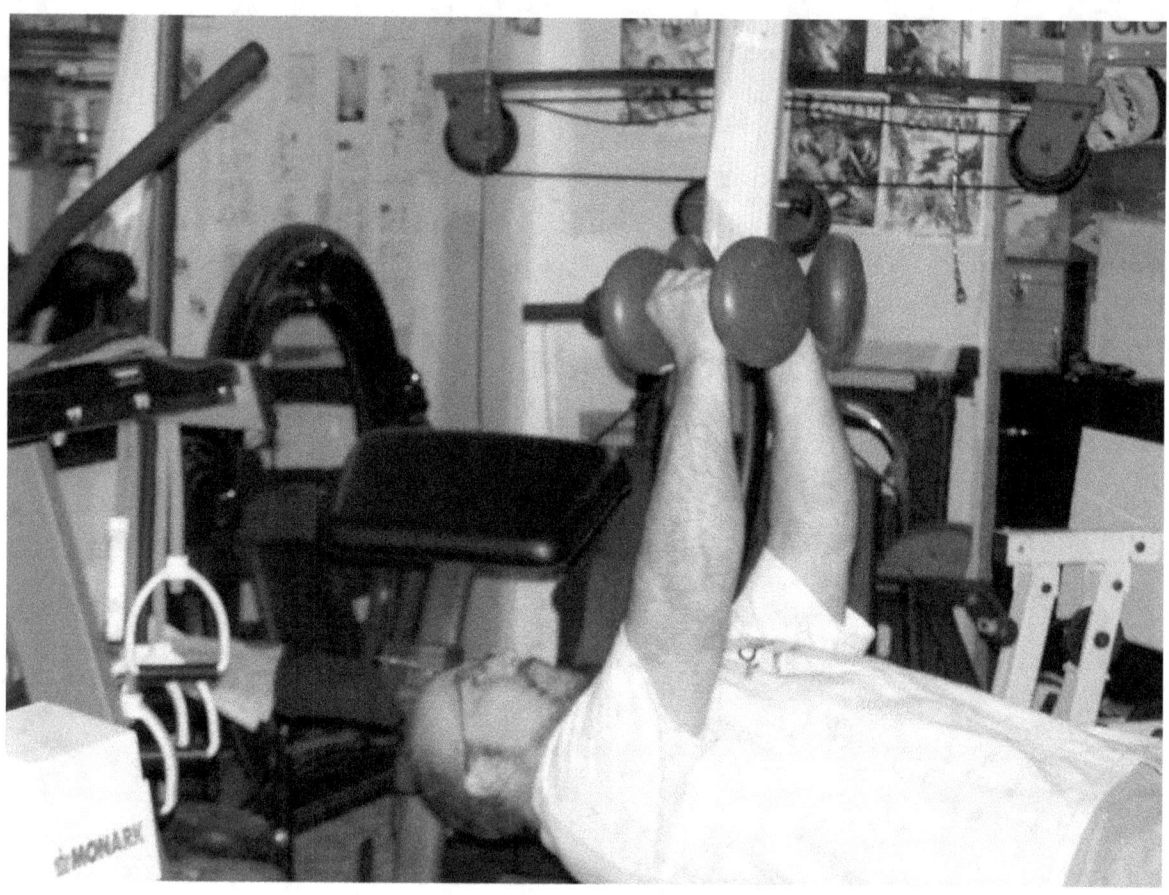

Pull

Tuesday

Squat or leg press (prefer squat), warm up first very light

Do 3 sets of 10-12 reps. do not break parallel with your legs.
Deadlift
Work up to 3 sets 10-12
Upper back, just 3 sets consisting of chin ups, 1 arm dumbbell rows, lat pull downs, seated rows; t-bar rows (pick 1 or 2)

Finish with biceps, 6 sets. Pick 1 or 2 of these; barbell curl, preacher curl, 1 arm seated alternate dumbbell curl, hammer curl, concentration curl.

Wednesday

Off except do some stretching and abdominal/ trunk work (crunches, sit-ups, leg lifts, trunk twists, your choice

Thursday

LIGHT version of Monday workout (60% Monday's weight)

Friday
LIGHT version of Tuesday's workout (60%)

Saturday
Similar to Wednesday

Sunday **REST**

You can change this around to have heavy push day on Monday and light pull day on Tuesday. You would then do light push day on Thursday, followed by heavy pull on Friday.

This is really a matter of preference and may work better for some.

Example 2

Fat burn, Tone-up routine

Monday:

Do 15 minutes total of calisthenics type moves and a couple of bodyweight strength/tone moves; Jumping jacks for 30 sec (need stopwatch or timer) rest 30 seconds, then do squat thrusts for 30 seconds, take 30 seconds rest. Lie on back, do Bike simulation, peddling in air 1 min, and then rest 30 seconds. Jump to feet, jog in place 1 minute, rest 30 seconds. Do abdominal crunches or leg lift for 30 seconds. Do pushups until failure point. Now, rest until your heart rate and breathing are at least close to back to normal, then repeat entire cycle. This whole thing should take around 15 minutes, but adjust times, rest periods according to your fitness level.

Tuesday:

Pick an item from the cardio menu, whichever you like. If you pick traditional, slower paced cardio, go at a moderate pace for at least 30 minutes, up to 1 hour (an hour is better). If you like the calisthenics type moves, you could choose to repeat yesterday's workout, or do a combination of the above.

Wednesday, repeat the Monday routine.
Thursday: REST

Friday, Sat, Sunday, repeat Monday, Tues, Wednesday cycle, then take a rest day,

Continue this cycle.

Example 3

For those who are in poor condition, very overweight or have a health condition:

Choose something from the cardio menu, like a slow walk. If you can walk (or swim, etc.) for 30 minutes without getting too exhausted, great. If you can't, do whatever is reasonable and comfortable at first, then gradually try to add a little time each workout. Ultimately, we want to build up to an hour. If that comes quickly, then just try to pick up the pace gradually.

Example 4

Beginner's mass/strength
(3 day routine)

Monday
Bench press, warm up well, then 3 sets 10-12
Dumbbell Fly 3sets 10-12 reps
Standing or seated overhead press, warm up, then 3sets 10-12
Dumbbell lateral raise 3 sets 10-12
Lying triceps extensions (or close grip bench press, about 8 inches apart0
5 sets 10-12
Abs 100 reps sit-ups, crunches, or whatever you like

Wed
Squat, warm up, then 3sets 10-12
Deadlift, warm up, then 3sets10-12 Abs, 100 reps again

Friday
Bench very light (60% of Mon weight)
Do bent over barbell rowing for upper back; Warm-up, then 3sets 10-12
Or Chin-ups if you have way to do
Do bicep curls , 5 or 6 sets of 10-12 reps, and abs again

Weekend off
If you need descriptions of exercises, go to EXRX or Bodybuilding.com website.
They have videos of about everything.
Give this a try to start, let me know how it goes,

Chapter 13

Periodization

This could be a sub chapter under "designing your program", but I thought it should be a chapter unto itself due to its importance.

There are various types of periodization or ways of practicing it. The most basic concept involved is that of progression. A typical weight training regimen is often referred to as a "**progressive resistance**" program. This just means the resistance should increase over a <u>period of time</u>..

One could also keep the actual resistance fixed, but increase the number of repetitions over a period of time.

The underlying problem with either of these scenarios is the dreaded "**plateau**" or "**sticking point**". This is when progress comes to a standstill in the routine, or comes close to that point.

When you exercise your muscles, you are actually breaking them down to some degree. In response, your body attempts to rebuild them just a little stronger so that they will be better suited to meet the demands that were recently placed on it.

Proper nutrition and rest are keys to how well this happens. Regardless of whether you are doing all the right things to recuperate and using proper training methods, your body's ability to adapt to new stress has its limits. **Sooner or later, doing the same routine continuously will fail to yield the desired results**. This is one of the big reasons people quit after a short time. New trainees usually make the best gains, and the body adapts relatively quickly for them. The more advanced level you reach, the more difficult it is to "trick" your body into making new adaptations and making gains.

Some people make gains easier than others, largely due to genetics, body type, etc. **Everybody can improve with training, regardless of where one starts out, and this is important to remember.**

Scientific studies on exercise have shown that trainees that have passed the new recruit phase typically only make good gains for the first 3 to 4 weeks of a new training program.

If we keep this in mind in designing our program, we can at least delay the onset of the plateau. In a perfect world, we should be able to avoid it altogether, but unfortunately, we don't live in a perfect world.

New trainees can easily do well at first by following a basic dual progressive system

This entails simply adding a repetition or 2 every other workout or so, then when you reach a pre-set number of repetitions, add weight and drop repetitions back to the original number again.
An example of this would be to start with 5 reps of 100 pounds in the bench press.
On the second or third workout, add a rep, or even 2 if possible.
Continue on in this fashion until reaching 10 reps with the hundred pounds.
Now, on the next workout, go up to 110 pounds, but go back to 5 reps, and then continue on adding a rep or 2 until you again reach 10 reps. If you can manage to add a rep every workout, great!
This is really another way of implementing the 3 steps forward, 2 steps back IDEA in different way. (Discussed in next section)

When you reach 10 reps with 100 pounds, going back to 5 reps with 110 pounds will really be going backwards in a sense, and should be very easy.

The idea is to allow yourself a break after making progress for a number of weeks, so that you can then start to rebuild momentum gradually.

The rookie can probably get away with cycling back only to 8 reps after a weight jump before restarting the repetition climbing routine.

3 Steps forward, 2 steps back

While many traditional progressive resistance programs have a form of periodization built in, it is not true periodization, really. For example, a traditional power routine for peaking one's strength for a competition would involve starting out with maybe 50 -60 % of one's 1 rep max lift, for 8 reps or so. The routine would probably suggest doing this for several weeks of gradually upping the weight to a higher percentage of the 1 rep max, and keeping the reps at 8 during that first few weeks. The next "phase" would involve dropping the repetitions to 5, and again progressively upping the weight over several weeks. This procedure is carried out further, until one is performing maximum single reps right before the competition.

The only thing you are really changing here is the rep scheme and weight used for those reps.

If you were to use the same weight on the week in which you drop the reps that you were using on the higher reps, this would be more like true periodization. Here is what I mean;

Week1   250x8, week 2 260x8, week 3 270x8   Now shift to sets of 5, but keep the first week at the same weight as your last set of 8's (270x5), now start adding weight as in phase 1 until you get to the next phase(sets of 3's.

The whole cycle would look something like this:

Phase 1 Week1 250x8's, wk2 260x8's, and wk3 270x8's

Phase 2 Wk1 270x5, wk2 280x5, wk3 290x5

Phase 3 Wk1 290x3, wk2 300x3, 310x3

Phase 4 wk1 310x1, wk2 320x1, wk3 330x1

This is just for illustration's sake. **The underlying principle here is that you back off right when a plateau would normally set in (3 weeks).** The body gets a break after it "peaks", and is able to recuperate and be ready for the next phase of progressive resistance advances.

Many trainees would actually add weight every week, including the week after the phase-shift, and in fact make a larger weight jump at that junction. The reasoning is that if you've just done 270 for 8 last week, and now you are dropping reps to 5, you should be easily able to do some extra weight, say 285 or 290x5 on this first workout of the new phase.

While this is completely true, it is **much more demanding on the body and therefore is difficult to sustain for any long multi-phase program, without using steroids or other potent ergogenic aids.**

The natural lifter would be wise to employ the periodization technique to promote longevity, avoid plateaus and prevent overuse injuries and injuries in general.

Another method of doing this concept would be to keep the rep number constant for longer, but rather than drop the reps on "week4" (really week 1 of new mini cycle), you would drop the poundage back to that done on the second workout and restart the progression. This is the 3 steps forward, 2 steps back routine as mentioned above.

You could perform a hybrid of the 2 concepts to peak for a competition. See the example below the chart given below for details on this. There are other ways of varying intensity and workloads, such as the more advanced level Russian concepts, where one does "speed training". This is based on percentage of 1 rep maximum. You would do 8 sets of 3 with 60% of 1RM, very explosively. You could then up the percentages gradually as you also lower reps to singles.

An alternative might be to use "speed training" one workout, alternating with a regular strength training workout on the other. (3 or 4 sets of 8s, 5's or whatever)

Some experimentation is really needed to find out which idea works the best for you.

Even when you find something that does work well; it is not likely to continue working forever without constant modifications and readjustments. The body is always adapting and changing, so the program musty follow suit.

I have seen so many guys that train very consistently and are pretty strong; however they fail to make real gains because they continue to do the same old tired routines. A famous person once said that **the definition of insanity is to do the same thing over and over and expect different results** (forgive me as I can't recall who said it)

Here is a table for calculating your 1 rep max for a given number of reps with a certain weight:

Simply go to the left column to find the weight used, move to the right until you are under the correct number of reps you are doing to find your 1 rep max. For example,

If you can do 10 reps with 205, you should be to do 1 rep with 267.

This is really just a rough guide and you may find it is either too optimistic or pessimistic in predicting your true 1 rep max.

This has to do with various things, like your fast-twitch to slow twitch muscle type ratio, skills in applying technique, etc.

I find I can usually max a little more than what is predicted on the chart, perhaps because I have more practice doing 1 rep singles being a powerlifter.

	2	3	4	5	6	7	8	9	
135	143	147	151	156	159	163	167	171	176
145	154	158	162	167	171	175	180	184	189
155	164	169	174	183	188	192	197	202	207
165	175	180	185	190	195	200	205	210	215
175	186	191	196	201	207	212	217	222	228
185	196	202	207	213	218	224	229	235	241

195	207	213	218	224	230	236	242	248	254
205	217	223	230	236	242	248	254	260	267
215	228	234	241	247	254	260	267	273	280
225	239	245	252	259	266	272	279	286	293
235	249	256	263	270	277	284	291	298	306
245	260	267	274	282	289	296	304	311	319
255	270	278	286	293	301	308	316	324	332
265	281	289	297	305	313	321	329	337	345
275	292	300	308	316	325	333	341	349	358
285	302	311	319	328	336	345	353	362	371
295	313	322	330	339	348	357	366	374	384
305	323	332	342	351	360	369	378	387	397
315	334	343	353	362	372	381	391	400	410
325	345	354	364	373	384	393	403	413	423
335	355	365	375	385	395	405	415	425	436
345	366	376	386	397	407	417	428	438	449
355	376	387	398	408	419	430	440	451	462
365	387	398	409	420	431	442	453	464	478
375	398	409	420	431	443	454	465	476	488
385	408	420	431	443	454	466	477	489	501
395	419	431	442	454	466	478	490	502	514
405	429	441	454	466	478	490	502	514	527
415	440	452	465	477	490	502	514	527	539
425	450	463	476	489	501	514	527	540	552
435	461	474	487	500	513	526	539	552	565
445	471	485	498	511	525	538	551	565	578
455	482	496	510	523	537	550	564	577	591
460	476	497	513	529	543	561	577	593	610
465	481	502	518	535	549	567	584	600	616
470	486	508	524	541	555	573	590	606	623

475	492	513	530	546	561	580	596	613	629
480	497	518	535	552	566	586	602	619	636
485	502	524	541	558	572	592	609	626	643
490	507	529	546	564	578	598	615	632	649
495	512	535	552	569	584	604	621	639	656
500	518	540	558	575	590	610	628	645	663
505	523	545	563	581	596	616	634	651	669
510	528	551	569	587	602	622	640	658	676
515	533	556	574	592	608	628	646	664	682
520	538	562	580	598	614	634	653	671	689
525	543	567	585	604	620	641	659	677	696
530	549	572	591	610	625	647	665	684	702
535	554	578	597	615	631	653	671	690	709
540	559	583	602	621	637	659	678	697	716
545	564	589	608	627	643	665	684	703	722
550	569	594	613	633	649	671	690	710	729
555	574	599	619	638	655	677	697	716	735
560	580	605	624	644	661	683	703	722	742
565	585	610	630	650	667	689	709	729	749
570	590	616	636	656	673	695	715	735	755
575	595	621	641	661	679	702	722	742	762
580	600	626	647	667	684	708	728	748	769
585	605	632	652	673	690	714	734	755	775
590	611	637	658	679	696	720	740	761	782
595	616	643	663	684	702	726	747	768	788
600	621	648	669	690	708	732	753	774	795
605	626	653	675	696	714	738	759	780	802
610	631	659	680	702	720	744	766	787	808
615	637	664	686	707	726	750	772	793	815
620	642	670	691	713	732	756	778	800	822

625	647	675	697	719	738	763	784	806	828
630	652	680	702	725	743	769	791	813	835
635	657	686	708	730	749	775	797	819	841
640	662	691	714	736	755	781	803	826	848
645	668	697	719	742	761	787	809	832	855
650	673	702	725	748	767	793	816	839	861
655	678	707	730	753	773	799	822	845	868
660	683	713	736	759	779	805	828	851	875
665	688	718	741	765	785	811	835	858	881
670	693	724	747	771	791	817	841	864	888
675	699	729	753	776	797	824	847	871	894
680	704	734	758	782	802	830	853	877	901
685	709	740	764	788	808	836	860	884	908
690	714	745	769	794	814	842	866	890	914
695	719	751	775	799	820	848	872	897	921
700	725	756	781	805	826	854	879	903	928
705	730	761	786	811	832	860	885	909	934
710	735	767	792	817	838	866	891	916	941
715	740	772	797	822	844	872	897	922	947
720	745	778	803	828	850	878	904	929	954
725	750	783	808	834	856	885	910	935	961
730	756	788	814	840	861	891	916	942	967
735	761	794	820	845	867	897	922	948	974
740	766	799	825	851	873	903	929	955	981
745	771	805	831	857	879	909	935	961	987
750	776	810	836	863	885	915	941	968	994

If you go by the chart and you follow my first example "periodized" routine, you would be starting out with a theoretical max of about 302, and finishing with a max of about 330. Not a bad gain for a 12 week program.

You would not be beat to death after it was over either.

If you were not training for a competition, you might want to follow a more traditional periodized routine in the 3 steps forward, 2 steps back format.

It would go something like this;

Week 1, 200x10's, week 2, 210 x 10's, week 3 220x10's (phase 1)

Week 4, 205x10's, week 5 215x10's, week 6 225x10's (phase 2)

Week 7, 215x8's, week8 225x8's, week 9 235x8's (phase 3)

Week 10, 225x 5's, week 11, 235x5's, week 12, 245x5's (phase 4)

If you refer again to the chart above, you will see that this program starts with a theoretical max of 254, and ends about 20 pounds higher after 12 weeks.

In theory, you could take a week in between your 12 week, 4 phase routines built like this, and end up with a very substantial rise in your 1 rep max after 1 t year (70-80 pounds.)

You could do this without ever doing less than 5 reps for the exercise in question, and with much less potential for injury and/or burnout.

This seems very easy to follow, but the most difficult part of doing it is to discipline yourself not to use more weight on the phase shift or "step-back week". This week should be easy, and it is tempting to add weight simply because it is not hard to do. It feels like you are going backwards rather than progressing, in the short term. You have to stay focused on the long term gains, which as you can see will come at the end of the program.

You don't have to follow this scheme for every individual exercise, but for at least the bench press, squat and Deadlift.

Also, this method is used more for a general mass and strength routine then if one is keying on trying to lose fat.

If you are trying to lose fat while toning up and adding some muscle, some of the keys are speed of total workout, strict form, and higher repetitions (8 or more reps at least)

You want to keep the heart rate elevated as in a cardio workout, but even higher than a typical "fat burning" cardio workout. Keep the time between sets very short, move quickly from 1 set to the next, do multi-joint type moves for the most part. Try to complete your workout in a set time period, and steadily try to improve that time.

Once you get the time cut down considerably, move the number of exercises up or maybe do 2 cycles of the same sequence of exercises that you have been doing.

The lose weight/ tone up example routine above is one way of doing this, but you could also substitute a circuit weight training type routine for the callisthenic routine, or develop your own hybrid of the two.

Just keep in mind if using the weights; you need to adjust the weights and reps to get the heart rate elevated above the normal fat burning target. You should be breathing pretty hard towards the end of your cycle.

If you start to hyperventilate, have trouble breathing, sweat profusely or have other symptoms of elevating your heart rate TOO high, then quickly "warm down" and stop the workout until you have fully recovered normal breathing.

Chapter 14

Spiritual Training

This chapter should really be chapter one, if I were following order of importance.
All of the physical training in the world will do nothing for your relationship with God, though some might claim this to be true.
Matthew 16:26 says:

For what is a man profited, if he shall gain the whole world, and lose his own soul? or what shall a man give in exchange for his soul?

In the same respect, if you become the strongest man or the fastest man or the best built man on earth, but lose your soul, what good is it? Obviously none!
Keeping spiritually fit requires discipline and a plan, like any fitness routine.

Like our body needs nutrients on a continual basis, our soul needs nutrients in terms of fellowship with other Christians, Bible reading/study, and prayer.

Get in the habit of daily bible reading and prayer, if you have not already done so.

It is good to setup a regular time for this if at all possible, but find a way to get it in.

I have a long commute back and forth to work. I listen to Christian radio programs, with preachers such as Charles Stanley, Chuck Swindoll, Adrian Rodgers and many others.

I pray every morning as I drive to work, at a minimum. You can talk to God anywhere, at any time, under any circumstances. If a crisis arises, say a quick prayer. If you hear some bad news, say a prayer.

Of course, there is a place for being alone in your room, on your knees, pouring your heart out to God, but that is not the only acceptable way to pray.

Some folks will say they don't need to attend church. They say that they can commune with God as they fish out in the woods, or they can watch a TV evangelist and get "fed" that way. To them I say "poppycock"

It is not only suggested in the Bible for us to have fellowship with each other, it is commanded!

1John 1:7 says:

But if we walk in the light, as he is in the light, we have fellowship one with another, and the blood of Jesus Christ his Son cleanseth us from all sin.

Matthew 18:20 says:

For where two or three are gathered together in My name, I am there in the midst of them."

Another good idea, other than attending regular Sunday church services, is to **attend prayer meetings or small group meetings if your church has these.**

Small groups can allow people to get to know each other and share each others joys and problems on a more intimate level than usually is possible at regular church services.

If you are not attending a good church on a regular basis, you need to make it a priority.

It can't be just any old church either. Make sure it is a gospel preaching church that believes in the Bible as the inerrant word of God, the virgin birth of Jesus Christ, The Trinity, the resurrection of Jesus Christ, the God-hood of Jesus Christ, and salvation by faith, not by works.

If you are having a problem with a specific area of sin, you must confess it of course, but sometimes having a fellow Christian keep you accountable can be of great help. It must be someone you can really trust, of course.

You must have Christian friends that you can confide in, hang out with, and talk to on a consistent basis, other than the formal church setting.

If you have unsaved friends, that's O.K., but if you attach yourself to them at the hip, your spiritual growth can't help but be affected negatively.

You don't have to do something "spiritual" every time you get together with Christians. Have fun! Go bowling, fishing, catch a ball game together, workout together, whatever. There are lots of resources for Christians online.

My church has downloadable sermons, as do many churches these days.

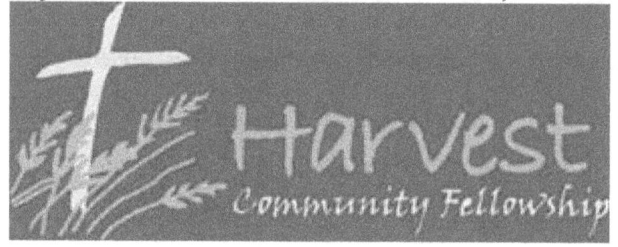

http://www.harvestcommunityfellowship.org/home.do

There are web-based Bible programs, like the Blue Letter Bible, which I use regularly.

http://www.blueletterbible.org/cgi-bin/tools/printer-friendly.pl?translation=NKJVP&book=Rev&chapter=19

The Fellowship of Christian Athletes, of which I am a member, has devotionals, interviews with Christian athletes and other great resources available online.

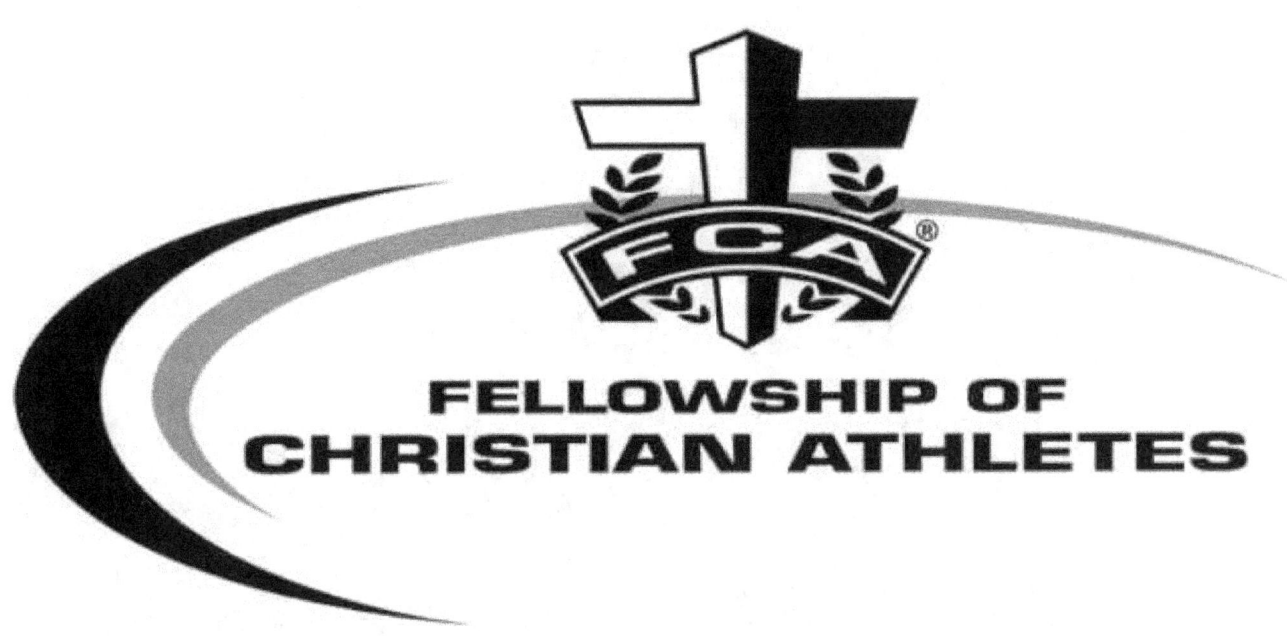

FELLOWSHIP OF CHRISTIAN ATHLETES

There are Christian discussion groups and forums, some strictly talking about faith issues, many others look at various aspects of life from a Christian viewpoint.

Here is one example

CrossDaily.com

http://forums.crossdaily.com/default.aspx

There is my **website   http:// Christianiron.com**, which is about fitness issues, training methods, etc., with a spiritual side.

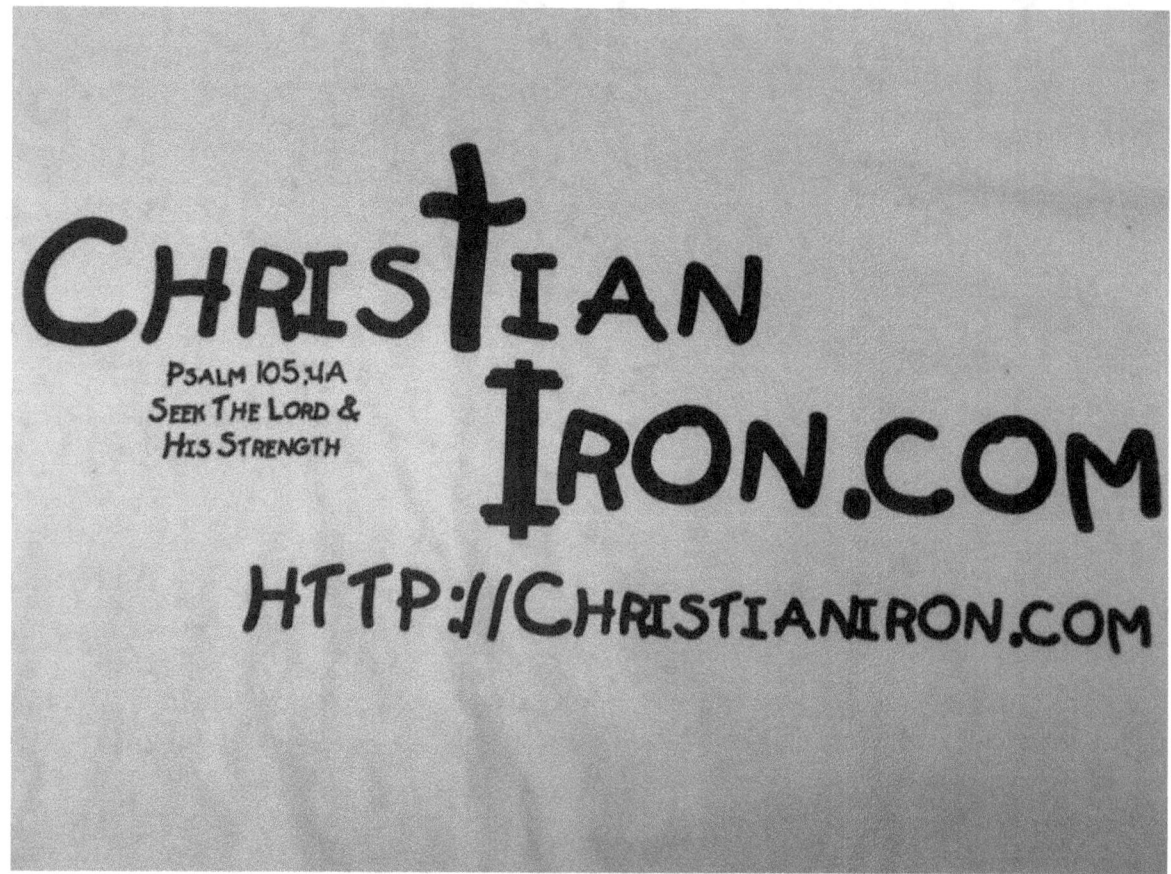

There are the Christian Powerlifters of America, of which I am also a member.

Christian Powerlifters of America

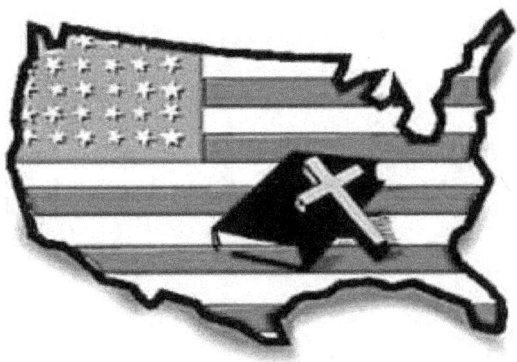

*"The LORD is my strength and my salvation; whom shall I fear?
the LORD is the strength of my life; of whom shall I be afraid?"*
Psalm 27:1

Here is a Christian Runner's website for those interested in running:

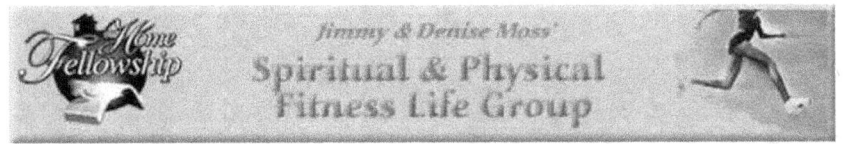

http://www.ourhomefellowship.com/jimmymoss.htm

If you look, you can find a group that shares your hobby or interest.

The Goal
Christian Sports of all kinds, testimonies, etc.

http://www.thegoal.com/

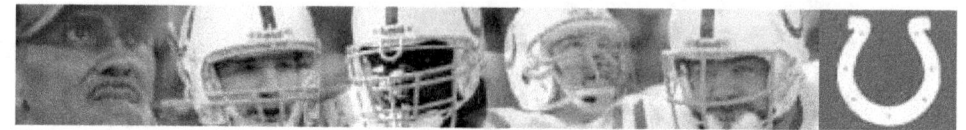

Above is a link to another nice Christian Sports site.

Here is a Christian Flag Football league

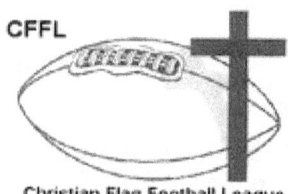

http://www.cffl.20m.com/index.html

Here are some Christian biking enthusiasts:

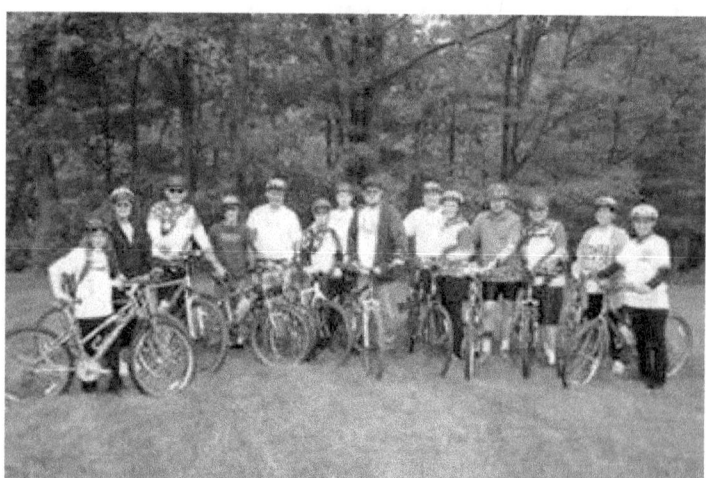

http://www.wheelpower.org/main/

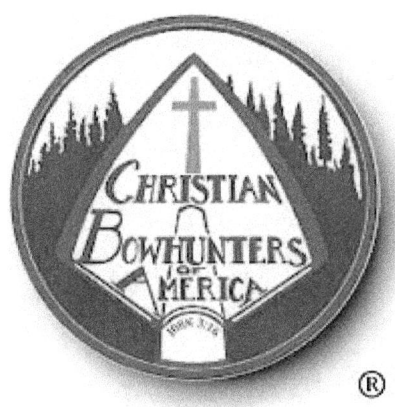

How about Christian Bow hunting?

http://www.christianbowhunters.org/

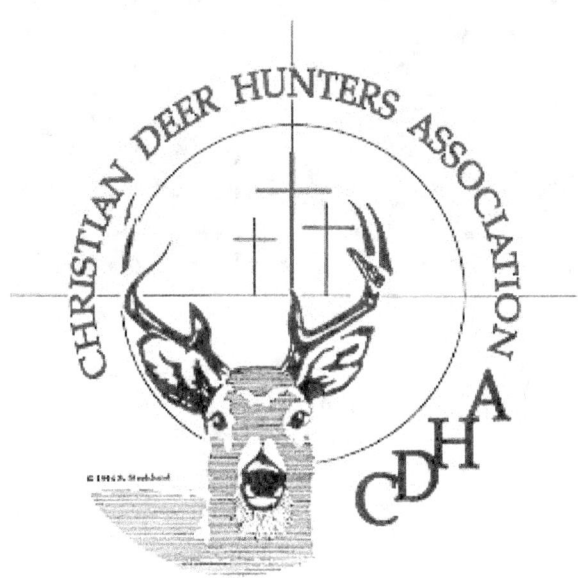

http://www.christiandeerhunters.org/

How about Christian Deer hunting in general?

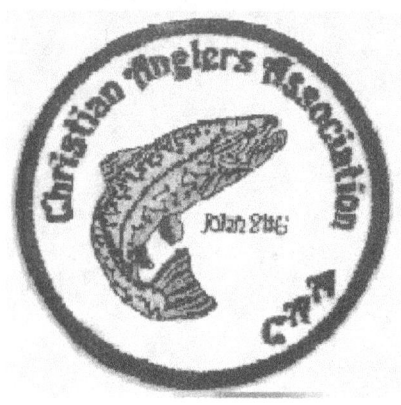

http://www.christiananglers.net/

Would you believe… Christian anglers?
The above outdoor sports are personally near to my heart!

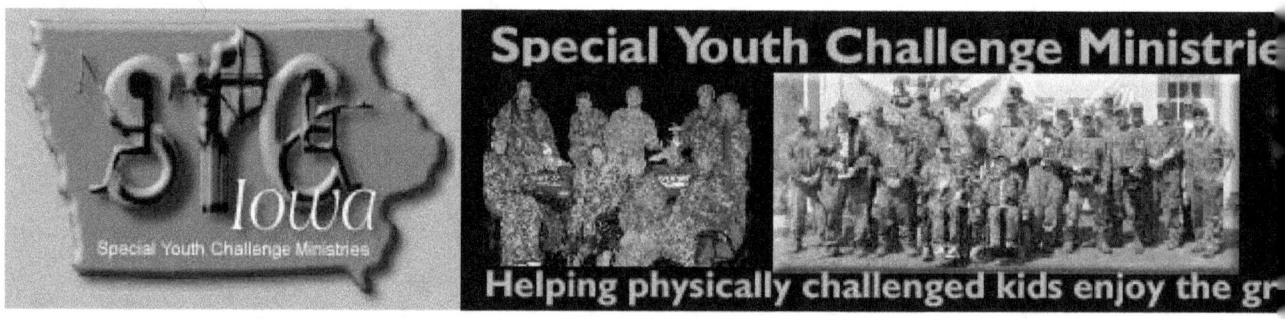

http://www.syciowa.com/

Here's a Christian Group that takes handicapped or underprivileged youngsters out for outdoor adventures!
The picture got cut off, but the last words are Iowa at the top, and outdoors at the bottom.

There are even ideas to **combine your spiritual and fitness training.** You can do a "prayer walk", where you take a walk on a regular path as you pray. (Not out loud, as you might find yourself in a straight jacket)
There are folks that practice a form of yoga, but in which they meditate on God and scripture instead of the standard mantra.
I'm sure there are others I have not come across yet.
There are other ways of integrating your spiritual life into other areas, like just being a good Christian example/witness at a competition.
You could wear a t-shirt with your church website, a Bible verse, etc. on it. We must certainly portray sportsmanship and the best of attitudes on the lifting platform, the track, or wherever we train or compete.

Family

Having devotions with the family is a great idea, but unfortunately one that has been largely abandoned by modern Christians. It's hard enough getting the family together for a meal, it seems.

In many ways, we have become too much like the world in the rearing of our children. I am not pointing fingers; I am very guilty of this myself. We really need to make time for our kids. Expecting them to get all the nurturing they need from school, even private school, and maybe a couple of hours of church attendance weekly just isn't going to cut it!

Men, we especially need to be examples and to help usher in our adolescent boys to manhood. This is a very critical point in their young lives, a time in which we could literally make them or break them.

They need our praise when they do well in any endeavor, and our affection on a regular basis (no, showing your boys affection is not effeminate)

They need validation that they have what it takes to be a man. If we call them ugly names, belittle artistic endeavors or things like this, we can really crush them and they may be scarred for life as a result of this.

Some of us try to live our lives vicariously through our kids, forcing them to engage in sports that we played or wanted to play, but that they are not really into.

Sports are good for kids, as long as they are enjoying themselves, it does not detract from other, more important aspects of their lives, and it's not overdone.

Chapter 15

Putting it all together

Well, at this point we've covered the exercise menu, nutrition, the mental aspect and more.

I've given some examples of exercise routines and how to use periodization in a program. We have talked about Spiritual fitness being incorporated into the program.
At this point, you should have some fairly good ideas that you intend to start working on. Many programs that have been written about or touted recently suggest large scale, radical changes that are expected to come about almost immediately.
I have no doubt that these programs will work for a lot of people, but perhaps are not for everyone. **Some folks need to work into the "lifestyle" in a more gradual, progressive fashion.**
This is, after all, something we want to make into **a lifestyle**; something we can do not just for the next 6, 12 weeks or even 6 months, but indefinitely.
While tremendous short term results with before and after testimonials are encouraging and uplifting, I wonder how many of these get fit quick stories end up as not so happily ever after endings.
What I would suggest, especially for those who have failed in diets and fitness routines in the past, or that don't feel an abundance of will power, is to **start small.**
Try to find the most pleasurable form of exercise you can stick with. **If one of the example programs seems insurmountable, scale it down to whatever you can comfortably do**. If you find that everything in the bad foods list is part of your regular diet, and few of the good ones are, don't try to pull an instant reverse. Instead, **try to remove an item from the bad list every day, or at least every week**. If your training regimen starts out as 10 minutes a day, up from zilch, that's O.K. to start with, as long as you try to add a little time on a regular basis until you hit the desired workout length (as in one of the examples.)
Nutritionally, I already mentioned that if you want to lose weight, **you must reduce calories and/or burn calories.** To gain, we must ad calories and do some muscle building exercises.
This sounds simple enough on its face, and is a mantra we have heard ad infinitum.
How do we know we are doing this if we don't really know how many calories we need or are presently consuming to maintain our current condition?
Various programs suggest actually tracking calories by using a scale, a calorie counting book, or something like this.
This is scientific and will work for those who employ it. **I don't think most people have the time or inclination to do this and this may be one more reason for folks to "fall off the wagon"**
I prefer to use the "keep it simple" approach in every aspect of life to which I can possibly apply it.
Accordingly, I think calorie counting is out for the majority of us.

Portion Control

Proverbs 23:21

For the drunkard and the glutton will come to poverty, and drowsiness will clothe [a man] with rags.

Portion control is a big factor, and one in which we as a nation have gone widely astray. This may be the biggest contributor to our obesity issues.

Restaurant portions have continued to grow in size over the years until they have become simply ludicrous in some situations. As youngsters, many of us were taught to **eat everything on our plate.** To do otherwise was considered wasteful, perhaps even unhealthy. We were even told we must clean our plates in order to get a desert, which contained even more sugar and fat.

We often stuff ourselves to the point of having to unbuckle our pants to relieve some pressure, both at restaurants and even at home.

Common sense should tell us this is not good portion control. Modern nutrition science tells us that **a "portion" of meat or fish or chicken is roughly the size of a deck of cards, or perhaps the size of the palm of your hand.**

A can of tuna or 6oz. piece of fish, chicken or meat is a reasonable portion for a single meal for the average person. If you read the label of a packaged food you are eating, it should give you the serving size, as well as how many servings are in the package. **We often mistakenly eat an entire package of something and consider it as a single serving, when in reality this is seldom the case.**

While I don't suggest counting every calorie you eat, **reading labels is a great idea.** You will learn what a serving size of your favorite snack is supposed to be, how much fat is in it, all kinds of things you may not have realized before. After a while, you will know what's in that package without having to read it every time.

A portion of protein with 2 portions of vegetables, fruits, pasta, legumes, rice or bread is a reasonable meal.

Multiple meals

Eating multiple meals throughout the day is **a good idea for several reasons.**
The first reason is that your **body is able to digest 5 or 6 smaller meals a day much better than 2 or 3 large ones.** The second reason is that your **metabolic rate will be speeded up,** because it actually takes some energy to process each meal. Finally, your **body will never go into "starvation alert mode".** This is where it starts to horde calories because it doesn't know when the next meal will be.
Never skip breakfast. The old adage that says breakfast is the most important meal of the day is very true. Skipping meals so that you can indulge yourself later on is a very bad idea, and simply does not work!
You can have 5 or 6 small meals, or you can have 3 bigger meals with a couple of snacks in between, just keep in mind that **snack doesn't mean junk**.
Of course, you can give yourself a break once in a while by indulging in whatever decadent food you crave. Having several slices of pizza once a week, or something along these lines, won't kill you. In fact, this will probably help you to stay motivated.
If you find yourself constantly going back for second helpings, or just not feeling full or satisfied after your plate full of food, there are some little things you can try that might help with this problem.
Try drinking a tall glass of water before a meal. You will get fuller, faster. Another idea is to **have a big salad before a meal**. Just avoid the croutons, bacon bits and heavy fat dressings. Some folks are great at taking an otherwise healthy salad and turning it into a gastronomical nightmare!
Eating a **salad with darker greens and adding lots of colorful veggies, with some light vinaigrette dressing is a great way to get the vitamins you need, has cancer fighting properties, and adds bulk without adding a lot of ugly calories.** It's not a bad idea to have a salad on a daily basis under any circumstances.
One other trick is to **use a smaller plate,** so that it appears to be piled with food.
I thought this idea to be kind of lame when I first encountered it, but data suggests it works at least for some.
Try some yogurt or salsa on top of your baked potato instead of butter or sour cream, or at least use non-fat sour cream if you must have it.

If you find yourself pressed for time and have a hard time finding enough time to get your workouts in as much as you might like to, there are some things you can do that may not come to mind immediately.
You can park a little further from the office or the store you are shopping at, and get in some extra walking. **Take the steps as opposed to the elevator or escalator when given the choice**. Get yourself one of those little pedometers to track your daily steps/miles. When you are more aware of this, it's easy to "kick it up a notch".

Take a walk during your lunch hour, or even get a quick workout in if you have facilities available.

If your workplace has a gym, try to get in a little early, get your workout in, take a quick shower, and you will feel energized and ready for the day!

Even if your workplace does not have a gym, perhaps they at least have a shower available.

You can get creative with the stairs at work and really get a good workout in by running up and down them, criss-crossing, skipping 2 or 3 steps in leaping bounds all the way up, etc.

You can walk, jog, jump rope, do calisthenics or similar things to get a workout in before work starts or during a break.

Use your imagination and have fun. Find a playground and do some gymnastic, bodyweight style exercises. Some folks are able to get in really good condition using these kinds of things instead of hitting the gym.

Play some ball with your kids, and get a workout while spending some quality time with them.

Do you suffer from arthritis, tendonitis or other joint problems? Try walking or working out in a pool, it's a lot more forgiving on the joints.

Look for ways to get around the obstacles. Don't make excuses for yourself, though there are plenty we can all come up with if we want to.

Always keep in mind; this is not an all or nothing proposition. 10 minutes of exercise is better than none. If you fall off the diet wagon, it's not the end of the world. Pick yourself up, brush yourself off and get back on the wagon.

Chapter 16

Advanced training techniques

In addition to the standard exercises in our menu, and following the periodization scheme of reps and sets, there are many other exercises and ways of performing them.

There are **supersets, giant sets, pyramids, split routines.** There is the muscle confusion concept, training to failure, pre-exhaust method, eccentrics, isometrics, isotonics, and the list goes on.

There is combat conditioning, strongman style training and boot camps of various kinds. You will hear about some of these concepts in the gym, on the internet, and in magazines and in other ways. While this is a primer, I would at least like to make you aware of some of these concepts, but I don't suggest you try them right away if you are a novice trainee.

Supersets

A superset is **simply 2 exercises done back to back, with no rest in between, usually for antagonistic muscles,** like biceps curls followed immediately with triceps extensions. You can do 3 exercises in a row, which would be a triset, or 4 or more which would become a giant set. These are very challenging and can **provide a tremendous pump effect.** They really get that lactic acid burn going. These are often done as part of a "cutting up" routine, where the trainee is seeking greater muscle definition, vascularity (Veins showing), and hardness, as opposed to building mass.

Pyramiding

This is a method of doing sets of lighter weight at higher repetitions, and gradually adding weight and cutting the repetitions down until one does 1 rep with a relatively high weight, and then going back down in the opposite fashion.
Alternatively, one could just do the positive side of the progression and stop at that, or vice-versa.
The concept behind this is that **one gets the benefits of the higher rep workout, like the pump effect, and the benefit of the heavier weight, low rep part being more beneficial for pure power, strength, and mass.**

The Pre-exhaustion technique

This method consists of doing some type of an isolation exercise for a body part that is also involved in the exercise to follow it. The second exercise will be a compound type of exercise as opposed to an isolation movement. For an example, you might do a triceps exercise followed by the bench press. The triceps contribute a lot to the bench press normally, but if you "pre-exhaust" the triceps muscle first, the bench press now has to rely much more on the pectoral and anterior deltoids to complete the repetitions, thus giving a heightened training effect for these muscles.

Eccentric sets

Every exercise consists of **a positive contraction, or shortening of the involved muscle(s), and then a negative "eccentric contraction" phase, in which the muscle lengthens back to its original starting condition.**
When using free weights, trainees often concentrate very heavily on the concentric phase and give little or no thought to the eccentric phase. This is unfortunate, as **the eccentric part of the movement may have even greater potential for causing growth than the concentric phase.**
You should always do the "negative" part of a movement with control. And not just allow the weight to drop back to the start position. That is just a more efficient way of performing any exercise repetition.
Beyond that however, **you can do an eccentric only phase of a lift with more weight than you could do the concentric phase with, and this is a way of stimulating growth beyond the normal set type.**
One might, for example, setup the bench press with about 120% of your 1 rep max weight, have 2 spotters assist you to unrack it, and simply bring it down, under control, to your chest. The spotters would then grab the weight and bring it back to the rack with little or no force from you.

This is not something that should be done frequently, as it really is effective in tearing down the muscle fibers, which is what a workout is supposed to do.

They are easily overdone and can lead quickly to overtraining. Extra recuperation time will probably be needed after one of these workouts, so be advised!

Forced reps

This method is exactly what it sounds like. **It is a way of extending a set beyond the normal failure point by having a spotter or 2 help finish an extra rep or 2.**
This is probably one of the most, if not the most overused and abused training methods there are.
Novice trainees should avoid this method, or at least use it very sparingly. I have seen too many trainees use a far too heavy weight, do an honest rep or 2, and have the spotter then assist in doing another 4, 5 or more reps. in this scenario; the spotter is getting more of a workout then the trainee. It is really ridiculous!
Used sparingly and wisely, it can be used to break through a plateau, but don't do more than 1 forced rep at the end of a set. Beyond that, you are basically wasting your time and your spotter's energy.

Cheat reps

Cheat reps are kind of **similar to forced reps with the exception that you can do them without a spotter.**

After performing a set in strict fashion and reaching the failure point, one could extend the set by using other body parts, letting form get "sloppy" or otherwise "cheating" a few more reps out of a set.

An example would be in the barbell curl. At the end of a strict set, one could swing the trunk of the body forward, then back to get some momentum, bending the legs just at the right moment also..
This is another highly overused method and its use can be the cause of injury if not done carefully.

Plyometrics

Plyometrics can be used even in less advanced routine, and in fact are **built into a typical aerobic step workout, to some degree**. If you play a game of hoops, you are really using Plyometrics when you jump as high as you can to make a rebound or take a jump shot. The key is an "**explosive**" movement, in which you are trying to generate as much force as possible in one burst. This can be as simple as a vertical jump from standing position, or a little more complex like jumping up on a box, then back down. One might also have a series of progressively higher boxes and jump from the lowest to each higher box consecutively. You could use a stairway for the same concept, taking 2 or 3 step "jumps" until you reach the top of the stairs. This is often done by athletes as part of their training to jump higher, longer, or perform other short bursts of powerful movements. Powerlifters and Olympic lifters incorporate these methods into their training as well. **Power equals strength x speed.**

Muscle Confusion

This idea just has to do with **changing the routine around constantly to avoid adaptation and plateau effects**. One might do giant sets in one workout, followed by a pyramid scheme on the next workout, and an eccentric workout on the third. This is used by advanced bodybuilders more than other type s of trainees. I am not crazy about it as it is hard to judge progress and I think it may have more potential for injury. That is just my gut feeling; I don't really have data to back it up. I suppose a little spat of this technique might help get you out of a "rut"

Strongman Type drills

Most of us have seen one of the "strongest man in the world" contests on television.
These types of competitions have filtered down to the local level these days, becoming a fun alternative to the typical powerlifting format.
There are a lot of different tests of strength and strength/endurance that are done at these events.
Lifting huge stones off the ground and placing them on a pillar, the "farmers walk",
Tossing huge tires around, carrying and throwing sandbags, pulling tremendous loads on a huge rope, and more are done at these events and as training for these events.
Pulling or pushing a weighted sled is another popular drill done not only by strongman competitors, but high school, college and pro footballers as well as powerlifters.
These types of events go beyond testing pure power, because stamina, speed and endurance also come into play in a big way, thus it's not always the biggest guys who win these competitions.
Another nice aspect of this type of training is that it **can be done very frugally**, using common household tools, implements and so forth. In fact, you could really make up your own strongman drills. Get some sandbags, ropes, big tires, sledgehammers, wheelbarrows, sleds or whatever else comes to mind and use your imagination.
You also get the added benefit of training outside when the weather is nice, which can really help in the motivational department.

Special Power building techniques

While old school powerlifting methods have always gotten results, there are many new wave techniques that have gained popularity these days, and many are used by the top handful of powerlifters in the world today.

The Russians have been building super athletes for years, and have excelled in producing very strong Olympic lifters and powerlifters and strongmen.

A lot of folks have chalked this up to steroid use as the primary cause, but this is not the full truth.

Russian Scientists have been experimenting with athletes and their training methods very intensely for many years and have accordingly developed **some tremendous training concepts and methods.**

They are big believers in using percentages of 1 rep max, as are many power trainers, but they tend to emphasize **speed training with relatively high volume, lower repetitions and lower weight**. Doing 8 sets of 3 reps with 65% of 1 rep max would be a typical early phase routine. Some trainees never even perform a single 1 rep maximum attempt before competing.

The concept is that once your reps slow down significantly, you are no longer training for power, but strength, since **speed is a major component of the power equation.**

Following this reasoning, doing explosive, fast reps with 65% of max is more efficient for building power than doing a slow grinding 1 rep 100% effort max lift.

Other techniques include **using bands and chains on the bar.** If you have heavy elastic bands attached from below the bar to the bar, the resistance overall will increase as the weight approaches the lockout or finish position. The same would be true with a heavy chain attached to the bar, with some or most of its weight lying on the floor at the starting position, and as the bar ascends the chains weight is added to the bar's weight.

As you might imagine**, this builds the lockout portion of a lift like nothing else can do**.

You can also do the reverse and emphasize the negative part of a lift by attaching bands to the bar from above.

An older method somewhat like this was the "stripping" method, in which spotters quickly remove weight from a loaded bar so that the lifter can then continue a set beyond the initial weight's failure point.

There are machines that do this for the lifter, without the need for spotters, and chains can be set up to do this method as well.

There are also special variations of more traditional movements, like zercher squats, Romanian deadlifts, and "benching" from the floor instead of a bench.

Box squats using various box heights also are highly used. **The reverse hyper is a relatively new machine that develops the glutes, hamstrings and lower back, said to add lots of weight to the trainee's deadlift and squat when used on a regular basis.** "**Rack work**" is really nothing new, but is also a special technique for working on just the "weak section" of a particular lift. For example, if one has problems with the lockout portion of the deadlift, one could set a very heavy weight up in the rack, with the pins set up just above the knees. Perform the lift just for that top few inches to build the lockout. There are more then mentioned here, but I just wanted to make you aware of some of the more popular methods that are being used. Again, most of these techniques are for the advanced lifter, not the novice or even intermediate lifter.

Chapter 17

Frugal Fitness

I have already touched on some of these ideas, but I wanted to make this a separate chapter as it is an area that is near and dear to my heart. Just ask my wife, I'm cheap! **It really does not have to cost a lot to workout; in fact, it doesn't have to cost anything if you really want to do it that way.**
I have searched high and wide for cheaper ways to workout, obtain equipment and get training info.
I have a pretty decently equipped home gym that I only spent a few hundred bucks putting together. **Thrift stores, yard sales, flea markets and the like offer fitness equipment that people are unloading at a big discount, often pennies on the dollar compared to buying new.**
Other places to look are eBay, Craigslist classifieds and your local newspaper or trading time's magazine.
Craigslist even has a freebie section, and unwanted fitness equipment can often be found there. (Just type craigslist classifieds into your search engine, it will come up)

You can choose to make your own equipment. I've found free online plans to build your own squat rack, benches, etc, out of wood, or if you have welding skills and equipment you can make some really heavy duty, super-sturdy stuff.

Here's a site that has lots of cool ideas:
http://www.angelfire.com/ny5/shenandoah/Grunt/grunt.html
(Grunt and Shen's Workshop)

If you can get some **large truck tires** for free somewhere, they can play a role in a combat conditioning or strongman style workout. **Sandbags** can be purchased cheaply or put together yourself even more cheaply.

You can **make your own medicine ball by taking an old soccer or volleyball, breaking it open, filling it with sand and putting back together**.
I actually made one recently using an old basketball filled with cat litter. It worked well, and it weighs about 12 pounds.

Here is another site with ideas for making your own kettle bell **handles on the cheap, how to make your own strongman yoke, farmer's walk apparatus, grip training ideas** and more:

http://www.geocities.com/fightraining/

Here is yet another:

http://www.davedraper.com/pmwiki/pmwiki.php/PmWiki/HomemadeEquipmentIdeas

Here is one with instructions for building your own **janda sit up machine** (extremely challenging), and other things:

http://geocities.com/briangl2002/index.htm

Here's one called the **starving student's power rack:**

http://redeye.co30.com/rack.html

Check out this site for real budget tricks:

http://jawbonejournal.blogspot.com/2007/04/debut-of-stonebell.html

Don't have weights or can't afford them?

Check this one out!
http://www.low-budget-warrior.com/Articles/AroundHouseWeights.doc

Along the lines of the site suggestions above, I took a couple of large tide laundry bottles that were destined for the trash or recycle bin, filled them with cat litter, and have a couple of 10 pound weather-proof weights for outdoor use.

Here is a blogger who uses pipes to make various pieces of equipment: http://makeyourowngear.blogspot.com/

You can take some PVC pieces and make a pair of pushup bars like the manufactured ones shown in a previous section of this book.

I already talked about using standard playground equipment to get in a good workout. **Monkey bars** can be hung from, you hand hand-walk on them, do pull-ups and chin-up variations, etc.
You can do rope climbing. You can grab the bottom of a swing seat and pull yourself up to it using the chain handles. (This is kind of an upside down pushup).
You can throw some weight plates in an old backpack and do your walking or jogging routines with some extra challenge.
You can do pushups with many variations, like one handed or clap pushups a la Rocky Balboa.
You could **fill a wheelbarrow** with any kind of weight, and push it up a hill a few times. See how long you can hold a heavy **sledgehammer**, extending it out with one hand.
Do the old family picnic favorite, the human wheelbarrow race, but put the backpack on the wheelbarrow for an added challenge.

I think I have given you enough ideas and places to find ideas here to really get your miserly juices flowing. Maybe you will have some ideas of your own after you take a good look at some of the sites I have suggested here.
There is no limit to what can be done for the creative person with some imagination! Have fun, which is what it's all about!

Free Training info

There is plenty of free training info available on the internet these days, but **you must not believe everything you see or hear ther**e. There is lots of miss-leading and bogus information out there along with the good stuff.

The library has plenty to offer, and is probably a more reliable source for quality information than random blogs and websites of self proclaimed gurus.

Cheap books and magazines can be picked up at some of the same places I mentioned in the section above on getting inexpensive used equipment.

There are some general rules to help you sift out some of the dross. **First of all, remember the old rule, if it sounds too good to be true, it almost certainly is too good to be true.**

Also beware of people selling a particular device or supplement that makes huge claims, but offers little but hype to support those claims.

Do yourself a big favor and read all you can about the fitness realm you want to involve yourself in.

Just like we are supposed to read our Bibles and know the content well in order to recognize false christs and false doctrines, we need to know as much as we can learn in the fitness areas so that we can recognize when something bogus pops up.

Please don't forget to check out my website at http://Christianiron.com. I offer lots of free info that you can either read online or download and read later. There are plenty of great links and more.

I also offer an email based "**virtual training service**" from the website which entails me setting up a training & diet regimen custom tailored to your needs and desires.

There is a monthly subscription to this service that you can opt out of anytime.

The price of a month's training is considerably less than the cost of the average in person session with a personal fitness trainer.

Your first, initial training consultation is free and will give you a good jump start.

You can stop there if you prefer, but I think you will find the regular consultations very helpful, at least for a couple of months as you start your program.